Who Cares?

AIDS in Africa

Susan S. Hunter

palgrave
macmillan

WHO CARES?
© Susan S. Hunter, 2003.

First published 2003 by
PALGRAVE MACMILLAN™
175 Fifth Avenue, New York, N.Y. 10010 and
Houndmills, Basingstoke, Hampshire, England RG21 6XS.
Companies and representatives throughout the world.

PALGRAVE MACMILLAN is the global academic imprint of the Palgrave Macmillan division of St. Martin's Press, LLC and of Palgrave Macmillan Ltd. Macmillan® is a registered trademark in the United States, United Kingdom and other countries. Palgrave is a registered trademark in the European Union and other countries.

ISBN 1–4039–3615–3 paperback

Library of Congress Cataloging-in-Publication Data
Hunter, Susan S.
    Who cares?: AIDS in Africa/by Susan Hunter.
        p. cm.
    Includes bibliographical references and index.
    ISBN 1–4039–3615–3
    AIDS (Disease)—Africa. I. Title.

RA643.86.A35H86 2003
362.1'969792'0096—dc22   2003055378

A catalogue record for this book is available from the British Library.

Design by Newgen Imaging systems (P) Ltd.

First edition: November 2003
10 9 8 7 6 5 4 3 2 1

Printed in the United States of America.

Contents

Preface

Many of my preliminary readers have said that they couldn't put this book down, that it reads like a novel, and that they loved the stories of Darwin and the courageous, unstoppable women in Africa who are committing small acts of heroism and kindness every day. If this book has one success, the one I wish for most is that it opens your heart to their struggle. It is for them that I undertook to write this book. In the distance I will always see them, the living heroes and the dead. In the fourteen years since I worked with the real "Molly," "Pauline," and "Robina" in Uganda, I have had the privilege of working with hundreds of other incredibly courageous people who are fighting this epidemic in Africa, Asia, Europe, the Caribbean, and the United States. Some are internationally known; hundreds more contribute to their countries, regions, or villages. Big or little, I have seen them perform miracles. Thank God for that.

My editor, Ella Pearce, is a bubbly, intense, articulate New York intellectual in her mid-twenties, who seems to waste no breath or motion. On our first meeting in the city, in February 2001, I got whiplash chasing her down the stairs of the Flatiron Building and across the street to the café where she informed me "all the editors take their writers." I almost choked when she said that, and I soon learned that Ella, flush with triumph after the publication of Peter Schwab's *Africa: A Continent Self-Destructs,* wanted me to write a layperson's book about HIV/AIDS in Africa. With her coaching, I submitted a proposal and spent close to eight months pulling together material on the book's many themes. A busy consulting schedule kept me from completing the first and very rough draft until January 2003. With Ella's help, the manuscript went through another four revisions. Talk about learning how to write! Thanks, Ella! It is a mark of her love for her writers that I never felt hassled, hurried, or browbeaten, a miracle considering how late I was with the initial manuscript.

The next person who deserves my undying gratitude is my friend, Gail Stern, who took on the task of editing my first book, *Reshaping Societies: HIV/AIDS and Social Change,* and as if that wasn't enough, muscled through the first and second versions of this book, giving me ideas and encouragement. It takes a very brave person to read through a rough draft. Thanks, Gail! The only other person brave enough to do that was Ella's Mom. Hopefully someday she'll meet my mother, Blanche Sefton, who read through a later version. The comments of my sisters, Margaret Bellucci and Joyce Devine, who read and commented on the final edit, were invaluable. The staff at Crandall library in Glens Falls, New York, were unflagging in their good cheer as they responded to one request after another. Thanks! And infinite thanks are due to Barbara Glaser, long-time friend and fellow board member of the Foundation for Hospices in Sub-Saharan Africa, who has stimulated my thinking, stood by my side, and pulled me out of a number of jams over the past many years. However, the fortitude of my dearest friend and husband Arlin Greene—whose specialty for more than twenty years has been jam-removal—cannot be compared with that of any other living mortal.

Friends and colleagues who were kind enough to read the final draft included Stephen Lewis, UN Secretary General Kofi Annan's special envoy on HIV/AIDS, who has been a sympathetic supporter since I first met him in 1998; Peter Piot, head of UNAIDS, with whom I've shared several podiums and whose encyclopedic knowledge and grasp of the danger of this disease always leave me stunned; Eric Sawyer, co-founder of ACT-UP and brilliant conceptualizer of the AIDS film, *A Closer Walk*; and Paul Zeitz, Executive Director of the Global AIDS Alliance and a tireless activist on the global AIDS scene who has been crucial in moving the world forward on a number of critical issues, including debt-for-AIDS relief.

Not everyone will agree with what I say. That is never possible. I only hope this book will fill a gap in the knowledge base, and that it will provoke controversy, study, counter arguments, and action. The Black Death that is AIDS in Africa deserves nothing less.

Lake Luzerne, New York
August 4, 2003

For my mother, Blanche Wronowski Sefton, whose Polish blood is my romantic-democratic wellspring.

And for my father, John Richard Sefton (1917 to 1994),
who died while I was in Africa.

CHAPTER ONE

Introduction

The early morning bustle of Kyotera town, in the heart of the Uganda's district of Rakai, had already begun. Radios blared, children cried, men called out to one another on their way to work, but Molly's warm brown eyes didn't snap open until daylight bounced off the rude stucco walls of her room and hit her chubby face. She was still tired after a restless sleep, but Molly knew she'd have to hurry this morning. The meeting with UK's Save the Children started at nine-thirty, and she had to remind Pauline to clean the reverend's shabby suit and make sure he wore his best dress collar before she ran over to the church hall to check on the lunch. Calvary Women's Group was cooking fish and *matooke*,[1] rice, and offal for one hundred people, no small job in the church's outdoor kitchen. She'd given Pauline the money to buy fish and banana yesterday, but they'd need plenty of firewood to get the rice boiled in time. She smiled with satisfaction. Something was finally going to happen.[2]

Robina Nyeko, the district administrator, had called the district-wide meeting so she could talk with Rakai's chiefs and subchiefs about creating volunteer village committees to look after the orphans, care for AIDS victims, and help stricken families as much as they could within their own small means. Parents were too ill to work, families were destitute, and dying was only a small part of their troubles. What she wouldn't give, Molly thought, for a little more help, as she watched these poor children grieve for their lost parents, abandoned by destitute relatives overloaded by the deaths of too many sons and daughters, helpless in a bad world. Yesterday she'd come upon Mrs. Kategera's five and seven year olds, who suffered through the long death of their father just last month, crying so hard she thought her heart would break. They'd worked all day on empty stomachs for the butcher,

Nsubuga, who'd asked them for twenty bundles of banana leaves to wrap his meat. When they brought him the last of it, he'd refused to pay, claiming to passersby that he simply didn't know why the children were bothering him for money.

Molly spotted Nina and Fabio being brutally embarrassed by the mean-spirited butcher in front of a growing crowd and ushered them away before they were blamed for any other wrongdoings. She was annoyed at the villagers for discouraging the children's determination, hard work, and inventiveness. They were ravenous after roaming the fields all day, but the tears spilling down their skinny, dirty cheeks dried into streaks as they ate their fill from Molly's cook pot. She walked them home so she could wash their mother, helpless in bed with AIDS, and clean the house up. Their one-room hut was badly in need of rethatching, Molly thought as they approached through the banana fields. Maybe she could persuade her brother-in-law to organize some men to get the roof fixed before the rains started again.

Molly greeted Mrs. Kategera, helped the emaciated woman up from her mat and walked with her out into the sunshine. She washed the diarrhea-stained sheets, hauled more water, gave the children and their mother a bath, and decided to clean their clothes while there was still enough daylight left to dry them. Mrs. Kategera's throat, full of thrush, was too sore for talk, but she smiled as Molly held her hand and told her how brave her children were, adding a few choice bits of village gossip to make her laugh. She'd found some old shorts for the boy but the little girl sat shivering, wrapped in the family's one tattered blanket until her dress dried. As Molly unsnarled the children's hair and braided it again, they began smiling too. Resilient, Molly thought. I hope it lasts.

As daylight waned, the children huddled close to their mother for warmth, and Molly stretched the thin blanket over their equally thin bodies. Taking Mrs. Kategera's clothes for washing, she stopped by the priest's house and asked him to alert the mission sisters. She feared for these children. What kind of people would they grow up to be if they were left on their own to cope? What would happen when their mother died? They had no relatives in the area because their parents had come across the border from Rwanda many years ago to work on one of Rakai's richest farms. Molly had made up her mind a long time ago that she would do all she could for people with AIDS and never give up hope. After days when it was all too much to bear, like yesterday, she'd cry herself to sleep, praying hard for some kind of inspiration.

Today it seemed like God had finally answered her prayers. November 3, 1989. She'd never forget the date. Molly rose and knelt by her small wood frame bed, glancing down at the foam mattress her husband had bought the year before he'd died. He'd said that they deserved a little luxury in their old age. Hard to believe, she thought, it's only been two years. Molly tried to decide which of her two worn blankets she would give to Nina and Fabio's mother, choosing the smaller one because it had the fewest holes. Then she closed her eyes and began. "Dear God," she prayed, "let this day go well. You've let the British see and know our struggles. Guide us to get more help for these children so they don't die of cold and hunger, sickness, and sadness. Let them know only your joy and not the harshness of life at such an early age. May you bring your judgment only upon the wicked of the world." Like that butcher Nsubuga, she thought.

"By the way, dear Lord, please help me find a job for Pauline's oldest son. His mother's sick and she can't afford the medicine." Pauline had been coughing up blood for at least two weeks, and Molly knew her tuberculosis was another symptom of her Slim Disease.[3] The ugly black scales were growing thicker on her face. "Six more orphans coming your way, Sweet Jesus, and it won't be very long now. Please remind these Save the Children people to bring a few extra blankets." Baby Jesus might have gone through a lot of things, she thought, but he'd never been an orphan. She crossed herself and rose. Pull up your socks, Molly girl, the day's only just begun. Don't start thinking too much about all these children. You'll drown.

Molly opened the door of her room just in time to see a parade of turkeys rush across the courtyard. They belonged to Mrs. Nyeko but wandered all over town. She called them "the Americans" because they reminded her of the new missionaries in Kyotera, rushing from here to there in a flock, scowling, busily inspecting things, very self-absorbed. She crossed to the outdoor toilet, shooing six enormous cockroaches away as she entered. When she was done, she went into the shower room she shared with twenty neighbors, removed her wrap, and drew cold water into a large flat basin. She soaped up, splashed the water over her back with a plastic cup to rinse, wrapped herself back up in her *katenge*, and crossed to her room to dress. Angela had already made up her bed and put a pink hibiscus flower and a spray of pine on her pillow. "Thank you, dear Lord," Molly said, "for all the small beauties you give us in this world."

Anxiety wrinkled Pauline's large, flat forehead as she waited for Molly to cross the road. Two bicycles were coming rapidly down the hill. Molly winced and lowered her eyes when she caught sight of the barkcloth-wrapped body strapped to the second man's back seat, rigid on a board sticking out on either side. "That'll be the second funeral in Nkebega's family in a year," Pauline muttered. "Those boys really liked their sex play," Molly agreed, "but if they'd had more sense on the black market, they'd be coming home in the back of a pickup truck." Pauline, a tall Ankole, laughed down at Molly, who was a short, fat barrel of a Ganda.[4] "Never blaspheme the dead," she chuckled. "As soon as you're finished in the kitchen, Mrs. Nyeko wants to see you. She needs help with the orphan report."

Molly had typed the orphan enumeration on Robina's prerevolutionary manual. There were 8,000 names in Kyotera alone, with four more counties still to be tabulated. Tough and seasoned to adversity, a great soldier and good administrator, Robina had sensed the tidal wave before anyone else had seen it coming. But it was Molly who'd suggested that she ask the chiefs, who had traditional responsibility for the welfare of village families, to list all their orphans. If they could demonstrate the awful impact of AIDS and the number of children that were being left behind, they might get some attention and help for Rakai, at least a little more than local communities could muster on their own. Deaths were such an everyday occurrence in the district that farmers had cut the grieving period from three days to one so they could still take care of their crops. The government had to be persuaded to stop ignoring the issue. The orphans in Luwero district created by Obote's genocidal purge in the mid-1980s were old news. Time the spotlight switched to Uganda's new tragedy, Molly thought, the day-to-day tragedy of AIDS.

⌘ ⌘ ⌘

On his return in 1836 from his five-year round-the-world voyage on the scientific ship HMS *Beagle*, Charles Darwin began to live two lives in earnest. In public he was an upstanding, hardworking, country-dwelling geologist. In private he harbored thoughts that would revolutionize the world. Darwin's voyage, scheduled for two years, had lasted almost five and yielded uncountable geologic and biological specimens and twenty-four densely packed notebooks of observations. To Darwin, the voyage had been "by far the most important event in my life"[5] and one for which his love of hunting, brief training in geological fieldwork, and greedy reading of travelogues and treatises in natural history had prepared him inadvertently but admirably. While purportedly studying medicine at Edinburgh University—before the brutal practice of the trade turned his stomach for good when he saw an operation on a child with no anesthetic—he had developed his lifelong passion for natural history. A lecture by John James Audubon on North American birds inspired him to study with John Edmonstone, a freed slave who had been taught taxidermy by his former master and supported himself mounting specimens for the university's natural history museum. An allowance from

Darwin's disapproving father, who had been persuaded by Darwin's uncle (and later father-in-law) Josiah Wedgwood that the voyage would prepare his son for the ministry, allowed Darwin to accept the loosely defined role of captain's companion and naturalist on the *Beagle*. It soon became one of history's most inspired volunteer assignments.

Freed for a while from economic concerns, Darwin could conduct scientific research to satisfy his curiosity, like other well-bred philosophers of the day. He also knew that his future income depended on the extent and quality of the specimens he collected on the voyage. Scientific curiosities were high entertainment for the Victorian public. The hummingbird collection of ornithologist John Gould, who later identified Darwin's bird specimens, was viewed by the royal family and crowds of commoners. The entrance fees for Gould's exhibit at the London zoological gardens paid his living expenses and financed later collecting expeditions. Darwin resolved that his own specimens would be worthy of "the largest & most central collection" in London, and he was right. Few scientists of the day had the opportunity to make a journey of similar length or scope or had Darwin's drive and experience in seeking out, preserving, and identifying specimens of great variety and comprehensiveness.

Darwin's letters home, published by the geologist Charles Lyell and fellow scientist Adam Sedgewick, and a brief showing of *Megatherium*[6] bones he had collected in Brazil's Bahía Blanca and shipped home in time for the British Association meeting in Cambridge in 1833, stirred public interest and excitement. On his return, Darwin was immediately named a fellow of the Geological Society and shortly thereafter a fellow of the Royal Society of London, science's highest honor. He had won his renown by five years of plain hard work, but now he had a bigger task in front of him. Publicly, that job was to edit thousands of pages of notebooks that he had kept on the voyage. Privately, he wanted to make sense of five years of flora, fauna, and people he had seen whose diversity did not fit with contemporary scientific theory. He devoted himself to the public task first, and *The Journal of Researches into the Geology and Natural History of the Various Countries Visited by H.M.S. Beagle* was published in 1839. The private task would take twenty years.

Although conscientious and dedicated, Darwin was a bold spirit. Since the *Beagle*'s movement made him seasick, he left the ship frequently to traverse hundreds of miles on foot and on horseback, joining the ship at its next port. Of his five years on the *Beagle*, only eighteen months were spent on board, and the longest stretch was forty-seven days. He fought his way out of the middle of armed political rebellions and enlisted the hardened gauchos of

Argentina, who joined him on long hunting and collecting expeditions, as staunch friends. Selected for the *Beagle*'s voyage because his upper-class background made him suitable company for the ship's captain, Robert Fitz Roy, Darwin nevertheless rolled up his sleeves to help the crew tow the ship's boats upstream on their river explorations and once even saved the *Beagle* from a tidal wave. Fitz Roy initially found Darwin's company so stimulating that he ignored Robert McCormick, the ship's official naturalist and surgeon. Annoyed by continual snubs, McCormick became so angry when the ship's carpenters began preparing packing cases for Darwin's first homebound shipment of specimens that he abandoned the *Beagle* at Rio less than four months after sailing from Plymouth, bought a souvenir parrot, and headed home (with Darwin's specimens) on the HMS *Tyne*.

Fitz Roy wanted Darwin to find scientific proof for the Book of Genesis. When he announced that the prehistoric *Megatherium* jawbone in Darwin's first load of fossils belonged to an animal that had been too slow to get on Noah's Ark, Darwin held his tongue. Struck by how much the gigantic prehistoric creature resembled South America's modern sloth, Darwin wondered why God had made the same species before and after the Flood. The idea that one could have evolved into the other because of environmental change seemed sensible to Darwin but theologically dangerous and scientifically absurd according to contemporary canon.

The *Beagle* carried three Tiera del Fuegians—York Minster, Fuegia Basket, and Jeremy Button—whom Fitz Roy had captured on an earlier voyage to the tip of South America. Fitz Roy had "civilized" them in England so they could proselytize their compatriots. Back on their native ground, the Fuegans quickly fell back into old ways, demoralizing the English parson who accompanied them so much he reboarded the *Beagle* as quickly as he could. The pathetic outcome of his inspired work put Fitz Roy in a black mood. Darwin's questioning of Christian orthodoxy and the Bible's creation story left Fitz Roy annoyed and unsettled, a grievously insulted host and sullen companion. During the four years and nine months of his voyage, Darwin revealed his deepest thoughts on geological, floral, and faunal change—"this wonderful relationship between the living and the dead" as he put it—only in his letters to Lyell, whose 1830 *Principles of Geology* argued that change in the earth's features had not required divine intervention but were the result of the natural forces of rain, wind, and erosion. Lyell's book had been Darwin's constant companion as he lay seasick in his hammock on the *Beagle*'s first leg south to Tenerife.

Darwin saw that as the environment changed, species had to change or they did not survive. Since environments had changed continuously on earth—evident to him from his inspection of the geological and biological record of "cataclysms" all around the world—species came and went, adapted or died. But what, he asked himself, was the mechanism of evolution? What drove the whole thing forward? Darwin gradually realized that one of the major forces in evolution was the force of disease. Humans evolve by adapting to disease, he knew, or they would die out just like any other species. This was an especially poignant realization for a man who complained in 1840 that he had become "a dull, old spiritless dog" at the age of thirty-one because of the chronic illness he had contracted in South America. He fretted to Lyell that "it is a bitter mortification to me to digest the conclusion that 'the race is for the strong' and that I shall probably do little but be content to admire the strides others make in science." Because of his persistence in the face of lifelong illness, however, Darwin became one of history's greatest scientists and his concept of evolution one of history's greatest ideas.

❊ ❊ ❊

HIV/AIDS is fast becoming the worst human disease disaster the world has ever seen. Although still in its infancy, it is clear now that in the next ten to fifteen years, AIDS will claim more lives than any other human epidemic ever recorded. Even if a cure is found tomorrow, AIDS is triggering a disaster worse than any the human race has ever known. By 2010, its death toll will be higher than that of the two world wars combined, and it will soon be worse than the total claimed by all wars put together. Every year and a half, it claims more human lives than the Holocaust, and with the pace accelerating, there will be a new holocaust every year. There is simply nothing left to compare it to, no scale of human suffering and devastation against which this terrible plague can possibly be measured. The global drag it has created is affecting every single human being on the planet without exception and is soon to get much, much worse as epidemics in Africa and Asia hit their stride. While infections in a few countries have leveled or are declining, in most countries HIV is spreading like wildfire. The 28 million deaths from AIDS at the end of 2002 are only a paltry beginning. It is little wonder that HIV/AIDS is the first disease to be labeled a global security threat by the United Nations Security Council, and the first disease to be the subject of an entire UN General Assembly meeting. At a November 2002 Washington dinner honoring UN Secretary General Kofi Annan for his diplomatic work in obtaining sanctions against Iraq, U.S. Secretary of State Colin Powell surprised the guests when he switched the focus from Baghdad and declared that the most serious problem facing the world today is not terrorism but the HIV/AIDS epidemic. AIDS is a not a future threat, it is destabilizing our entire planet right now and will have far worse consequences than any event a terrorist could ever invent.

While the story of Darwin's professional career and personal life in the mid-1800s and the story of the small-town Ugandans Molly, Pauline, and Robina are more than a hundred years and many miles apart, they are united by the underlying theme of humans needing to explain and respond to widespread disease, to the changes epidemics make in human communities, and how these responses shape the evolution of the human species. As we follow both of their stories in this book, we will also be looking at the facts behind the AIDS epidemic, at how other epidemics have shaped world history, and at evolutionary trends in sexuality and disease. But Darwin, Molly, Pauline, and Robina are key to our understanding of AIDS because the scientific and social stories behind the HIV/AIDS epidemic and the relationship of evolution and disease it exemplifies are profoundly personal stories, histories of struggle with a stern and terrible disease that will change our very future as a human race more than any war or act of terrorism ever could.

As we follow Darwin on his life's odyssey, we will learn more about how he gave birth to the idea of evolution, one of the most important ideas in the history of thought, an idea that has shaped all of human and biological science since he first announced it in 1859. We will see how that idea has improved public health, medical science, and response to epidemics, and how it also has been misused to justify the oppression and deprivation of human beings thought to be inferior on the scale of social evolution or marginal to its course. In Darwin we will find a profoundly empathetic and gentle human being who opposed racism and slavery in all its forms, a courageous man who put forward an enormously unpopular idea at a time when stern prejudices were used to control "deviant," "immoral," and unsettling thoughts and actions. In Darwin we will find an adventurer, a keen observer of life in all its forms, and a lively painter of human realities and geological marvels that helped to educate his Victorian public. And we will find a demure and retiring family man, a loving and gentle spouse, whose loss of two children shaped his vision of the human condition and the role of God in human affairs.

At the same time, we will follow Molly, Pauline, and Robina as they shape one of the first community responses to HIV/AIDS in the late 1980s in Uganda, the first African country to be badly hurt by this global epidemic. We will take a close look at the history of Africa, key to understanding who our Ugandan women are, the challenges they face, and how they formulate their responses and worldviews and hold onto their faith and goodwill during these times of ultimate loss. We will be taking a look at key factors that have played a role in African development and in forging the continent's relationship to the rest of the world, and at the devastating consequence of colonialism in Africa and elsewhere, because these experiences have shaped the disease histories of all developing world regions. The ideas of community solidarity and self-help that inspired the work of Molly, Pauline, and Robina in Uganda quickly spread to other countries in eastern and southern Africa and now inspire community-based HIV/AIDS work all over sub-Saharan Africa and in all countries with serious HIV/AIDS epidemics. They inspire and inform work in hard-hit communities of Asia, the Caribbean, and Latin America, and have been carried by African social workers and public health experts to Baltimore and New York, where they were used as the basis for developing community-based responses to AIDS in metropolitan settings.

This book is more comprehensive than the typical AIDS book because it is premised on the idea that we have to widen our focus from the relatively narrow fields of science and medicine to look at the epidemic's social, political, and historical antecedents if we are going to find a "cure" for AIDS. We have a lot to learn from taking a close look at past epidemics, especially those of sexually transmitted diseases (STDs), and from evolutionary insights into human sexual and social behavior. HIV/AIDS in Africa is particularly illustrative of many of these converging themes, so while HIV continues to spread in other parts of the world at a dizzying rate, uncontained by the best medical and public health minds, this book takes Africa as its focus. It is no accident that HIV/AIDS has spread there with such overwhelming and pitiless consequences and that currently Africa has three-quarters of the world's HIV/AIDS burden. But the situation is likely to be as bad or worse in Asia and Russia over the next ten to fifteen years, so Africa can teach us a lot if we are willing to learn.

By taking a closer, more reasoned look at why Africa has failed to develop as a continent, we can understand the future of AIDS on other continents. Africa is only the worst case of an inhumane scenario being played out in other regions of the world to the detriment of the human species as a whole. The growing wealth of developed countries over the past two centuries and the growing impoverishment of developing regions are inescapably related. The deprivation that limits the lives of one in every five human beings on the planet creates a burden of moral responsibility not only to give back, but to think about a strategy that yields a safer and saner world for the children of every country in the twenty-first century. As HIV/AIDS and other epidemic diseases increase, they are creating a huge disease reservoir that threatens the very existence of humankind. One of the most important evolutionary relationships is between humans and their microbes, and many scientists feel that because of fundamental neglect of the needs of 20 percent of the human race, the microbes are winning.

The emergence of HIV/AIDS late in the twentieth century would not have surprised Darwin very much, any more than it surprises modern evolutionary biologists. Darwin would have been dismayed at the role played by more than a century of misinterpretation of his notion of survival of the fittest—its use as a weapon against some members of the human species by others—and would have spoken resoundingly against it. The emergence of HIV/AIDS in Africa is a result of the convergence of long-developing trends in human history, technology, philosophy, and evolution. Social, political, and economic trends set afoot in Darwin's time and justified by his theories have played themselves out with earth-shattering consequences, producing just the sort of results he feared the most.

The sense of urgency created by the rapid spread of HIV/AIDS across sub-Saharan Africa and its continued escalation in other parts of the developing world is well deserved. According to Dr. David Morens of the University of Hawaii and National Institutes of Health, the news is not good. When seen from Darwin's perspective—from the point of view of evolution—"humans are standing at the edge of disaster. There are already 6 billion people on our planet, and the global population continues to grow at a great rate. Our societies haven't imploded yet only because most of the world lives at a level of privation Westerners would not accept, beyond the reach of the very resources Westerners cannot live without."[7] As one small example, the Netherlands sustains itself by drawing off the resources of an area fifteen times its actual size, which British disease ecologist Tony McMichael characterizes as a "subsidy," realized from the resource flows that rich countries established from the 1500s through the 1960s, during hundreds of years of colonial rule. Our longer life expectancies are another measure of the benefits of the wealth we have acquired from the environmental resources of other less powerful populations by "borrowing," as McMichael phrases it, "against the environmental capital of future generations."[8]

The poor countries of the world suffer, among other things, higher rates of illness and shorter life expectancies as a result of this borrowing, and McMichael thinks that "in an increasingly unequal world (where the several hundred richest individuals today have a combined income equal to the world's poorest 3 billion people) one must conclude that the global economy is, in some ways, acting to the detriment of the health of large parts of the human population."[9] The global HIV/AIDS pandemic has come at a time when new findings in human biological and social evolution are converging, causing us to question and expand traditional views of disease and its agents, forcing us to restate our understanding of the relationship of human and natural agency in shaping epidemics. We are forced to reconsider our notion of ethics and of what we might owe to those same people of Africa whose demise plays itself out before our very eyes. "Back to Africa" leader Marcus Garvey's exclamation after World War I that "if the West Africans had not been there, the Kaiser would be sitting in Buckingham Palace" was no hyperbole.[10]

A successful response by the human race to the HIV/AIDS epidemic must, in the end, be composed of equal parts of science and economics and serious humanitarian concern for our future. AIDS may be the toughest challenge we've ever had to face, stretching our capacity to feel as well as think, our ability to balance scientific genius and economic considerations with our fundamental humanity in the face of human suffering and loss. The response must be measured in small steps and little ways, in acts of kindness and salvation by ordinary people, as much as it is in the giant steps of Nobel Prize-winning ingenuity.

The question of what to do about HIV/AIDS in Africa will not be resolved by science alone. We already know at least nine ways to prevent further spread of the disease and how to respond to its victims. While a vaccine could avert total global disaster, it is far in the future and a little beside the point. We can stop this disease with prevention and treatment but hesitate because of the cost. What faces us now are questions of morality, the same questions that Darwin wrestled with as he thought about the implications of his new evolutionary theory. Darwin's connections to God had become so attenuated by scientific inquiry his wife worried that he had become an atheist and would suffer God's eternal punishment for his doubts, but he strongly believed that God, although distant, had not abandoned the world entirely. Where in the rough-and-tumble, often cruel world, Darwin wondered, did God fit in? Where in our own rough-and-tumble twenty-first century do morality, ethics, and human sensitivity to suffering and pain fit in? Where, in the modern dilemma of AIDS, do we weigh in as individuals and as countries?

Certainly, so far, *not* on the side of the angels. Our feet are planted firmly on the ground as we create more and more ways to study AIDS but few ways to address it. Scientists are lost in the numbers: medical researchers search for a cure; historians document AIDS in Africa as another result of colonial and cold war privation; economists look for "cost-effective" ways to stop it. As we procrastinate, women like Molly, Robina, and Pauline are learning to address their holocaust, facing the incredible odds of their struggle with clarity, perceptiveness, and humanity, with no place to turn but their faith—and their pluck, inventiveness, creativity, and intelligence. While our minds are lost in heady debates over AIDS numbers and lofty HIV theory, their feet are tripping and stumbling over the bodies and, in some areas of Africa, literally running out of places to bury them. The question of what to do with those bodies—already 28 million in number and soon to mount to over 100 million—must plague our thoughts and wills.

By learning more about the epidemic and its causes in poverty in the developing world we can guide our politicians to make better decisions. Before we look into African development, the history of epidemics, human sexuality and the coevolution of humans and their diseases, let us take a longer look at the HIV/AIDS epidemic itself. In chapter 2, we will take a look at how far and fast HIV/AIDS has spread, the effects it is having, and how it can be prevented, detected, and treated. African development, a mine-field of moral implications as well as a fascinating story of human action and beliefs, follows in chapter 3. The history of epidemic diseases around the world, the subject of chapter 4, is a story more of failures than successes, but in chapter 5 we will see how more effective responses have been gradually for-mulated by the human race. Even in the case of STDs, raging around the world since the 1400s and the subject of chapter 6, humans were able, over the last one hundred years, to find effective responses. Responses to disease are key determinants of the course of human evolution, and as we will see in chapter 7, we may be losing the war with our microbes. In chapter 8, we will confront some of the political and economic factors shaping our lack of response to AIDS and what this means for our future as a species.

Our track record with STDs is especially interesting because it shows how the potential scientific effectiveness of prevention and treatment became a victim of the same "moral" issues that hinder effective responses to HIV/AIDS today. But the story of syphilis also can give us hope, because it shows how we can be successful in combating an STD in a relatively short time when we face it squarely. We desperately need to learn from our past, because HIV is only the most dangerous STD we now face. Other STDs are proliferating, causing widespread infertility and leading to undetected but serious chronic physical and mental deterioration in their carriers all over the world.

Unless we act, the future is not bright. Although medical science responded rapidly in the early stages of the AIDS epidemic, progress in developing a cure or a vaccine has come to something of a standstill. In fact, halfway through the world's most promising vaccine trials, the disease mutated and recombined, forcing stunned scientists to modify the vaccine and hope for the best.[11] Besides an impressive ability to mutate, AIDS may behave like other epidemic diseases have in the past, mutating like syphilis did in the 1500s, taking other internal and external forms, and switching the manner in which it is transmitted. Imagine, for a moment, if AIDS became a respiratory infection and could be transmitted by a sneeze like the bubonic plague did when it became the Black Death in 1347. "No rule of nature contradicts such a possibility," says Joshua Lederberg, former president of Rockefeller University. "The proliferation of AIDS cases with secondary pneumonia multiplies the odds of such a mutant, as an analogue to the emergence of pneumonic plague."[12]

Long-term control of the disease requires individual and social change, a coming to maturity of our personal and social ethics, the commanding of personal sexual urges, and reduction of deep-seated addictions usually acquired in adolescence. Even when AIDS grows out of a small reservoir of drug addicts, its spread into the larger population capitalizes on the human drive for sex, our most fundamental biological urge to re-create ourselves as a species. Since HIV/AIDS is about sex, we must learn to speak clearly and without shame so we can be more frank about protecting our young people. Curbing the epidemic also requires governmental behavior change and change in economic systems, both of which seem to be as slow in coming as individual change. Above all, it requires a paradigm shift, the kind of change human beings find hardest to make, a change in our basic understanding of how things work, an acknowledgment of how deeply and intricately all systems of this earth are intertwined in ways much more subtle than our intellect is able to comprehend. Arriving at that kind of paradigm change requires a fundamental honesty, looking at and responding to the world as it really is. Darwin had that kind of honesty, lack of pretense, and curiosity. He spoke of the delicate web connecting all living beings in mysterious and unpredictable ways with a real humility that most of us have forgotten. It is the humility and honesty that animates ongoing community-based responses to HIV/AIDS in Uganda and around the world. Let us go back and see how Molly, Pauline, and Robina are doing. But first a little story from my own time in Africa, where I lived from 1989 to 1995.

�֍ ✖ ✖

It's been raining for forty days and forty nights here in Kampala—at least that is what it feels like. The rain hasn't stopped for what seems like weeks here in the capital of Uganda, a little country astride the equator famous in history for the martyr of twelve small boys, early Christian converts who would not submit to the king's insistence on a night of lust and became Africa's first saints. The Pearl of Africa, Uganda was called, the jewel of British East African colonies, whose seven hills of Kampala blush with the spill of bougainvillea and poinsettia and every other conceivable flowering miracle. In Uganda, they say that if you push a stick into the ground, it will blossom and bear fruit. Kampala is home to Makerere University, where British and American students came to get their master's degrees in the 1960s and 1970s. Seven years later, it was headquarters for Idi Amin's terror factory in the Nile Hotel, not a mile from the Makerere. In the 1980s, Uganda was the first country in sub-Saharan Africa to be hit hard by the AIDS epidemic and one of the first countries to control it.

I'm here in the early morning of liberation, just as the air clears from the smoke of battle, on the first day of 1989. Teaching at Makerere, that once famous university where Amin's son, desperate for the attention he could not possibly receive academically, raised hell with women and shot holes in his dorm room ceiling. The school collapsed into ruin during Uganda's long years of war. Books were stolen for to wrap fish in the market. Every electric socket and bulb—any exposed wiring at all—was ripped from the wall. A university with no books, desks, paper, computers, or students. We've had seven strikes since I started teaching in early March and it's now May 1. For the most part, the strikes were nonviolent, but later in May two students will be shot when the president sends in the tanks. For now, just me and a few other lecturers, here only when they are not out busy making money someplace else.

I share a house, a wonderful old university professor's two-story stucco monster that must have been the bee's knees in its day, with leaking roof and oh-so-wonderful long open living room-dining room combination where we have the occasional pizza party when we can get cheese. My roommate and I have a wonderful maid, Medina, named for the city of Mohammed's birth. She is one of Uganda's 2 million Muslims, more, Quadafi once said, than in all of Libya. Medina is chocolate-brown, in her early thirties, and has dimples that never tire. She is entirely self-reliant, raising seven children on her own. Two, Douglas and David, are Irish twins, six and seven years old. There's only one after that—the pediatrician across the street helped Medina get her tubes tied before she suffered uterine collapse, the most common reason for female hospital admissions in Uganda.

It's raining, sheets of rain pouring off the roof, so I've decided to spend the day at home reading and planning my lectures. I'm making lunch in the back kitchen and stick my head out the door to make sure I'm still here on the planet, and there they are, Douglas and David, dry under the overhanging eaves. Dry, and working away with such quiet intensity that they barely notice my presence. There, spread between them, is a complete marching band and an entire sitting orchestra—ah, the miracles of Africa!—made out of mud. Each figure is recognizable, each instrument modeled to perfection, each tiny hand fingering a note. And each one four inches tall, if that, no more. Red mud in the hands of geniuses who had only glimpsed the university marching band at the recent graduation or seen, one time, a photograph of an orchestra in a magazine.

I draw in my breath. If there is any miracle in Africa, this is it.

CHAPTER TWO

AIDS and the World

Molly's favorite musician, Philly Lutaaya, was just thirty-two when he returned to Uganda in 1989 from a recording session in Sweden and announced that he had AIDS. A native son who had entertained in European and African capitals, Philly went public when he was relatively healthy so that fellow Ugandans would become more aware of the disease. Philly, like most African men his age, took it as a given that he would never sleep alone if he could possibly help it, and his fame had made him attractive to women far and wide. When Philly got AIDS, Molly, like most Ugandans, refused to believe it. He looked well when he first came home, leading many to believe that he was pulling a publicity stunt. When he "turned eighty" less than three months later, Molly had the satisfaction of collecting on a small bet from Pauline, who was much more cynical about everything, not just Molly's beloved Philly.

"Look at the poor man," Molly said. "His hair has fallen out, he's lost half his weight, he needs help walking because of the foot fungus, and he can barely sing." "Not the first one I've seen," Pauline snorted. "Just the most famous. And if he thinks he can keep these young men from their sex play by opening his mouth to show off that ugly white stuff he's got growing in it,[1] he's hallucinating." Molly hummed the first few bars of Lutaaya's *Alone and Frightened*[2]: "Today it's me, tomorrow someone else, let's fight together in the war against AIDS," and Pauline joined her, singing as they walked across town to call on Robina. During Philly's last visit to Masaka, when he'd come to visit his family and traveled to Rakai to warn young people to "love carefully," Molly was inspired by the idea that each village in the district should list its orphans so the impact of AIDS would be known.

"I hope this orphan count doesn't turn out like the time you volunteered on the mission's pediatric ward," Pauline teased her. "Life is for the living," Molly replied. "There were three or four children huddled in every bed, skinny as sticks. Some had even been left on the floor because there weren't any more beds. Their mothers rocked them all the time, but they cried and cried and cried. Rashes, diarrhea, pneumonia. The mothers' torment never ended because there was no medicine to relieve the children's suffering. The death bell rang at least twice an hour and finally I couldn't stand it any longer." Pauline stopped in her tracks. "It's so frustrating to know that rich people in Uganda and other places spend millions on their own care but have nothing to share with these poor women,"she said. Like you before long, Molly thought.

"This time," Molly said, "we'll be helping kids that still have a chance. I just hope this meeting isn't like the last one." Pauline laughed so hard she had to stop again. "Do you remember when the young chief from Kabula tried to eat his own pencil the whole time Robina was talking about helping the children? I thought that British woman would die of a heart attack." "It certainly strained all her good manners not to stare at him, but I don't think she heard much of what was being said," Molly replied. "When Slim hits your brain," Pauline said, "it sure does funny things. Such a shame in such a handsome young man. The only way I could refuse him sex when he asked me later was to tell him my husband was coming home." "You don't have a husband!" Molly laughed. "Not anymore," Pauline sniffed. "He even offered me some money. I almost went for it when he pulled out the bills, but I just knew it was trouble all around. Sarah's school fees are due and we haven't had any sugar for weeks." "I saw him later with that girl from Lyantonde," Molly told her. "She can't be any older than fourteen," Pauline gasped. "That may be true, but I know she didn't refuse," Molly said, "and her mother was standing right there. These Ganda women are too well trained. They think they can't refuse a man, and they definitely didn't know he has AIDS. He looks normal, except when he's pushing a pencil. Too darn ignorant. That's what happens when schools are closed for fifteen years."

❊ ❊ ❊

Darwin's *Journal of the Voyages* was so popular among amateur naturalists and scientists alike that it quickly sold out its first print run. His readers compared him to a painter who had the power to make them see, hear, smell, and feel places they could never hope to visit themselves. Baron Alexander von Humboldt, the greatest scientific explorer of the age—whose travelogue of the Canary Islands, South America, Mexico, and the United States from 1790 to 1804 inspired Darwin to learn Spanish the year before he began his voyage—found Darwin's descriptions "happily inspired" and Darwin an "eloquent interpreter of nature's facts." In Bahía, the *Beagle*'s first Brazilian port of call, even a torrential rainfall had not diminished Darwin's spirits. "I can only add raptures to the former raptures... each new valley is more beautiful than the last." Perched on a log in the lush tropical forest, he wrote that "delight is a weak term to express the feelings of a naturalist who for the first time has wandered by himself in a Brazilian forest... [it] bewilders the mind." His Bahía adventures were soon topped by his explorations of the wild Argentina pampas, sailing in the dangerous Strait of Magellan, and climbing the high mountain of Chile.

Darwin learned from the little as well as the big, from tiny creatures as well as the fossilized remains of giant prehistoric animals. Even the dust from the air collecting on the *Beagle*'s deck 300 miles from land was a subject for study. Germany's C. G. Ehrenberg, one of the leading microscopists of the day, found sixty-seven different organic forms in five packets of dust Darwin sent from off the coast of Cape Verde, all of them different from the African samples Ehrenberg had analyzed previously. Disease-causing microbes were just being identified in Darwin's day, and his experiments showed that even these tiniest of creatures could travel the globe as easily as he could.

Traveling south along the coast of Argentina, Darwin woke one night and, disentangling his feet from the chest of drawers where he stuck them when sleeping, rolled out of the hammock he unfurled over the ship's chart table to make his way to the rear deck of the 90-foot *Beagle*. It pitched in high seas as the vessel plunged through the open ocean, but Darwin grabbed tightly to the rail, drawn toward the front of the ship by a ghastly, entrancing glow. "There was a fresh breeze," he wrote, "and every part of the surface... now glowed with a pale light. The vessel drove before her bows billows of liquid phosphorus, and in her wake she was followed by a milky train. As far as the eye reached, the crest of every wave was bright, and the sky above the horizon, from the reflected glare of these livid flames, was not so utterly obscure as over the vault of the heavens." Study of Ehrenberg's work told Darwin that these particles were living beings whose phosphorescence remained long after they had died. When he agitated them in a tumbler, they gave out sparks, white or green depending on the minute living beings within.

In Darwin's first published note about natural variation, he describes a Cape Verde kingfisher perched on a castor oil plant, pecking at lizards and grasshoppers. It "was brightly coloured, but not so beautiful as the European species; in its flight, manners, and place of habitation, which is generally in the driest valley, there is also a wide difference." On the Galapagos Islands, his growing concept of adaptation was reaffirmed when he saw that each island had its own unique set of birds, lizards, and even giant tortoises. They resembled South American species but were not exactly the same. Back in England, he enlisted the help of his children in experiments to prove that plant seeds could be carried thousands of miles in the ocean or deposited in the droppings of sea birds to show how South American species came to the Galapagos.

Darwin made friends with native people easily, admiring and observing them as closely as he did the landscape. One evening in Ribiera Grande, a small town east of Porto Praya, Cape Verde, he wrote that the locals, "all as black as jet," watched them eat dinner and how "everything we said or did was followed by their hearty laughter." Of Fuetes, a tiny village on a small stream, he wrote that "everything appeared to prosper well, excepting, indeed, that which ought to do so most—its inhabitants. The black children, completely naked, and looking very wretched, were carrying bundles of fire-wood half as big as their bodies." He knew that the rough appearance and demeanor of the Argentine gauchos did not diminish the accomplishments of men as proficient in their world as he was in his. Seeing the man Tierra del Fuegan Jeremy Button had become when Captain Fitz Roy took him to England—and the man he was reduced to upon his return to the harsh land-scape of his home where his adaptation to English society meant little—gave Darwin direct insight into the vast adaptive capacity of human beings.

Darwin's experiences were unique in the Victorian world. Only one of his contemporaries, his friend, correspondent, and rival Alfred Russel Wallace, had a similar breadth of experience and intellect. Seeing the world in all its vastness, splendor, and variety helped these two Victorian naturalists realize that earlier speculations about change in the natural world, including those of Darwin's own grandfather, Erasmus, were right. God had not created and re-created each living and fossil species over and over again. They had created themselves by adapting to the conditions around them. Like scientists today, Darwin enlisted the help of all the great minds of his day, a whole consortium of collaborating scientists helped him interpret his specimens when he returned. In addition to Ehrenberg, they included John Stephens Henslow, who had taught him botany as a professor at Cambridge and recommended him to Fitz Roy, the zoologist William Whewell, ornithologist (and hummingbird exhibitor) John Gould, and Richard Owen (who would later become his arch rival) to interpret his fossils.

✼ ✼ ✼

The creative tension of scientific competition and collaboration has been as important in advancing the science of HIV/AIDS as it was to the spinning of evolutionary theory in Darwin's day. In only twenty years, since the first AIDS case was diagnosed in 1982, scientists identified the human immun-odeficiency virus (HIV) responsible for autoimmune deficiency disease, or AIDS, developed blood tests to diagnose the disease, and engineered treatments to extend the life of the infected. This is the first time we have had the capacity to watch a massive, global disease event unfold before our very eyes and the first time we had the means to change an epidemic's course before it became a global scourge. Although repeated waves of many other diseases— plague, influenza, tuberculosis, cholera, syphilis—have swept the world since the turn of the twentieth century, HIV/AIDS is the first epidemic of *a totally new disease* since the 1400s. It is the first global epidemic to begin after medicine crossed the threshold to modernity in the 1950s, gaining the laboratory capability to identify a disease and its causes quickly, the field capacity to prevent its spread, and the data systems needed to track epidemic growth virtually as it occurs. HIV/AIDS is the leading infectious disease threat in the world today, outpacing the two next most important infectious diseases, tuberculosis and malaria, two to one. Not only is it the leading killer in many developing countries, but in the early 1990s it established an early lead over older diseases to become the leading cause of death among eighteen- to thirty-four-year-olds in the United States, where it is now the third leading cause of death among all age groups and rising once again.[3]

HIV, the virus that causes AIDS after lying quiet in an individual for seven to ten years, currently infects 42 million people worldwide.[4] By the end of 2002, the disease had already killed 28 million people, and an estimated 3 million people now die from the disease each year. This is 8,200 per day, almost three times the number who died in the World Trade Center attack on September 11, 2001. In total, more than 70 million people worldwide have been infected by HIV since the first cases were recorded in 1982 and at least 5 million additional people are being infected each year—some 15,000 per day. If these rates remain the same through the first decade of the twenty-first century, at least 52 million people will have died by 2010 and 58 million will be alive but infected with the virus.

It is likely, given recent reports of infected blood transfusions in China and the HIV mushroom cloud in India and Russia, that global infection rates will soar even higher. An assessment by the U.S. National Intelligence Council in September 2002 warns that the infected populations of five countries alone—Nigeria, Ethiopia, Russia, India, and China—will be 75 million by 2010.[5] If they are added to the existing global HIV reservoir, by 2010 at the very minimum 130 million people will be "incubators walking around with this virus, spreading it to other people," according to Gary Nable, director of the U.S. Vaccine Research Center. Environmentalists warn that South Africa, where one-fifth of adults are HIV-positive, is facing a cemetery crisis and environmental disaster because more than 3 million bodies must be buried over the next ten years. The country's Town and Regional Planning Commission says that with 16,000 people dying each day countrywide, the equivalent of 3,240 football fields will be needed to accommodate the dead in Kwa Zulu Natal Province alone.

AIDS surpassed the Black Death's total carnage of 25 million in Europe by the end of 2001 but has not yet topped the *global* death toll from the Black Death, which swept across China, India, the Middle East, and northern Africa before it tainted the wind in Florence in 1347, killing one-quarter to one-half of the inhabitants of every world region except the Americas.[6] It will do so by 2010, when the AIDS death toll will also easily surpass the world's next largest historical disease catastrophe, the depopulation of the Americas in the early 1500s. HIV/AIDS is at least ten times deadlier than any war on the planet and will soon outdistance any of the world's most deadly twentieth-century conflicts.[7] World War I and II together killed 60 million people, the war in Vietnam, 5.1 million combatants and civilians, and the conflict in Korea, 2.4 million. By 2010, if HIV rates remain the same, AIDS will take almost as many lives as those conflicts *plus* the U.S. Civil War, the Bolshevik Revolution, the first Chinese communist war, the Spanish Civil War, the Taiping Rebellion, the Great War in La Plata, and the partition of India put together.

If we count those who are dying *each day*, AIDS is three times more deadly than terrorism. If we count total number infected *each day*, it is five times more lethal. The disease is a pervasive security threat because it leads to growing poverty, food insecurity, economic and social collapse, deaths among the armed forces and police, increased criminal violence, and sudden power imbalances. In 1990 Kenneth Kaunda, then Zambian president, told a visiting U.S. Congressman that he did not know what he would do when the population of street children in that country's capital, Lusaka, reached 500,000 because the roaming bands of uneducated and unsocialized orphans would become uncontrollable. The U.S. Central Intelligence Agency called AIDS a security threat in 1999, and in January 2001 a National Intelligence Counsel report warned of massive loss of military capabilities and a 20 percent drop in sub-Saharan Africa's gross domestic product (GDP) in less than ten years. Countries in the region may not be able to uphold their peacekeeping commitments on the continent because of mounting deaths. In reverse, of course, war, chaos, economic uncertainty, and social disruption create the perfect conditions for rapid disease spread.

The problem is not just in Africa. From a handful of cases reported in the United States, Europe, and Africa in the early 1980s, AIDS has spread to millions of people in every country of the world. When it first developed, many parts of the world were "clean." By 1993 Poland, countries in Southeast Asia, and Greenland—formerly "clean" areas—reported infections, and by the turn of the twenty-first century there was not an infection-free state in the world. HIV/AIDS is fast becoming the biggest disease burden in the world. Measured by premature death, loss of human potential, disability, and by diminishing capacity and siphoning off scarce resources, HIV/AIDS creates losses for everyone, infected or not. Disastrous socioeconomic consequences are predicted for Eurasia as well. The American Enterprise Institute's Nicholas Eberstadt projects huge death tolls, failed economic growth, and dangerous political imbalances in China, India, and Russia by 2025 as a result of AIDS.[8]

Global drag is created because in countries where 20 to 40 percent of the population is infected and 60 percent of new infections occur in people under age twenty-four, AIDS not only kills the most productive people in a society, but they pull others down with them as they slowly and inexorably die. HIV/AIDS deaths and illnesses create huge demographic gaps and vast political, economic, and social problems while it kills off the very people who can address them. The growing food crisis in southern Africa over the past few years is due in large part to HIV/AIDS, which has reduced productivity while increasing the number of desperate individuals who are willing to violate social rules to get food and meet other social needs. Recent food emergencies in that region have put 14.4 million people at risk of starvation, in part because 7 million agricultural workers have died from AIDS since 1985.

※ ※ ※

Although people are living longer with HIV than they were when the disease was first identified in the 1980s, death from AIDS is usually a difficult and prolonged affair. "As I traveled from orphanages in Africa to hospices in Russia to clinics in Thailand," one reporter wrote, "I saw the tortured face of AIDS. It grimaced with the pain of fever and nausea. It gasped with fluid-filled lungs. It wore huge, open sores that emerged from deep in the throat and spread over the lips, neck, and torso. In advanced stages of the disease, the central nervous system can begin to deteriorate, leaving some victims powerless even to close their eyes and mouths. Nerve endings in the extremities go numb or tingle as if pricked by thousands of needles. AIDS robs the brain of its cognitive functions, leaving patients raving with dementia. It saps the body's protein, wasting muscles to the bone. Even the release of death can lie weeks or months away." AIDS has created millions of Philly Lutaayas, twenty- to thirty-year-olds who turn old overnight and waste away rapidly, skeletons draped in nothing but skin. HIV erodes the body's defense system, exposing the infected person to a range of lung diseases, cancers, fungal infections, diarrhea, wasting, rashes, sores, and other painful and debilitating conditions. Eventually these AIDS-related illnesses overpower the body's ability to fight back, causing physical—and sometimes mental—ruin and death. There is no cure for AIDS, but antiretrovirals extend life by slowing the progression of HIV. Opportunistic infections that kill nine of ten AIDS sufferers also can be treated, but most of the necessary drugs are unaffordable in developing countries.

As a pathogenic agent, HIV is ideal because it has virtually no external symptoms for seven to ten years. Ninety-five percent of HIV-positive people around the world feel healthy, do not get tested, and easily and unwittingly pass the virus on to wives, husbands, partners, and friends. Of the five ways HIV is usually contracted, ordinary heterosexual intercourse is the most common, with homosexual or bisexual intercourse and injecting drug use in second and third place. HIV generally starts in a core group of people with a high infection rate—like sex workers or drug users sharing needles—and quickly fans out to the wider group of people with whom they have contact—their customers, spouses, children—people with ordinary lifestyles and no "high risk" behavior of their own. The fourth transmission route, from mother to child *in utero* and during birth and breast-feeding, means that 30 percent of the babies born to HIV-positive mothers will be positive unless a brief, easy, and cheap preventive therapy with antiretrovirals is provided.

The last transmission route is through infected blood transfusions or blood products, like those used by hemophiliacs. Since the first blood bank scare in the United States in the early 1980s, countries have tried to protect, with varying degrees of success, the safety of their blood supply. African countries struggled to maintain a clean blood supply with declining resources throughout the 1990s and still have trouble doing so not because of technical reasons but because countries are too poor to purchase enough test kits. Belief that a country is not threatened by HIV has also delayed implementation of safety measures in a number of Asian countries. In 2002 a catastrophe in China, where at least 1 million poor Chinese—some believe the figure is closer to 10 million—donating blood so they could buy food were infected by faulty transfusion methods, shows how dangerous this sense of isolation can be.

Two driving forces in rapid HIV/AIDS spread, poverty and labor migration, are not sexual at all but lead ordinary people into behavior that places them at risk for HIV infection. From the karaoke bars in Dongguan, China—a hub of global manufacturing just inland from Hong Kong, where sleek, tall Mongolian girls bounce on the laps of squat Taiwanese business-men who do not let the fact that they have had one two many sticky wines interfere with their ability to bellow "to dream the impossible dream" at the top of their lungs—to the sleepy township bars surrounding South African gold and platinum mines that turn into steamy hot spots for sexual liaison at night, male and female labor migrants in developing countries leave their families behind for months and years at a time in order to feed and provide for them.[9] A large proportion of female migrants are kidnapped or lured into the sex trade on the promise of a better-paying job in the city, or work for predatory employers even farther away from home in order to provide their children the essentials. For more than a century, more than 1 million migrants to South Africa's Witwatersrand, the heart of the country's gold mining industry, have carried sexually transmitted diseases home to other parts of the continent. The mines now employ 300,000 workers on yearly contracts away from their wives and families, and their "long absences from home, the tedious, dangerous work, the drab anomie of life in all-male min-ers' hostels, the gangs of prostitutes clinging to the chain link fences around the mines" have contributed to the rapid spread of HIV in South Africa and all of its neighboring countries.[10]

The phenomenon is not unique to Africa. Waiting in Ha Noi emigration lines to board a return flight to United States, I learn from the man behind me that he is headed for Perth, Australia, to join an uncle with an established laundry business. "No work Vietnam," he grins, what few teeth he has left gleaming black in his skinny face. While he is typical of the more than 170 million people around the globe who do not live in the country of their birth, migrants are "highly atypical," generally more adventurous and less fearful than those who do not migrate. Developed countries, where one of every ten people is a migrant, receive 2.3 million newcomers from less-developed regions each year, accounting for more than two-thirds of their annual population growth. While almost half of all developed countries try to bar less-skilled immigrants, third world countries are routinely robbed of their doctors, nurses, engineers, and scientists. The outlook for teachers is very bright; over the next ten years more than half the teachers in the United States will retire, keeping foreign recruiting firms busy finding 2 million replacements to meet rising student enrollments. The economic value of these mass movements is an extraordinary $73 billion in remittances each year, money sent home to waiting families that amounts to 10 percent or more of the GDP of at least nine countries. Even more people migrate within their own countries each year, but their movements are less well documented.

A key factor in the spread of all global epidemics, migration has played a huge role in spreading HIV from place to place from the epidemic's start. Canadian air steward Gaetan Dugas, HIV/AIDS's "Patient 0," infected at least 40 of the first 248 gay men diagnosed with the disease in the United States. Dugas had at least 2,500 sexual partners in the ten years he criss-crossed the United States and Canada, leaving a deadly good-bye gift for each and every one, but only forty were definitely traced.[11] Official and illegal migrants cross borders, grab planes, and jump on ferry boats to get to desperately needed work. Most of the migrants spreading HIV—men traveling to large job sites in construction, manufacturing, or mining, and the women who follow them, as well as teachers, doctors, nurses, nannies, and computer consultants—are not anywhere near as sexually active as Dugas. They do not have to be to catch HIV, which typically infects 50 to 90 percent of the sex workers in a developing country unless they are registered and treated by the government. Infected migrants take HIV home to their entire families with no partner the wiser until one gets sick or a baby is born that does not thrive. The nineteen-year-old wife of a migrant who regularly leaves his home in western Mexico's rural El Fuerte to go to the United States to work, where she knows he visits sex workers, says that it would be a breach of trust to ask him to use a condom when he gets home. "You can't really prevent it," she says of HIV, "you just have to believe him." Another woman remarks that "AIDS is really spreading in Mexico because many men whose wives are in Mexico [go to the United States] and get involved with someone, and they don't know if she has AIDS. Then they get it, and they go back to Mexico."[12]

Another type of migrant—working on short-term maneuvers, stationed for longer periods at border outposts, fighting full-fledged wars, or manning peacekeeping missions—is the soldier. Throughout recorded history, soldiers have been an enormously successful "vector" for disease transmission, and many of the world's armies now have HIV infection rates that are two to five times higher than the general population. Two decades of fighting in Angola, for example, have left it "a lethally perfect Petri dish for HIV," where demobilized troops believe that sex with a virgin or herbal remedies cure AIDS, condoms cause impotence, and young women cannot contract the disease. According to the Center for International and Strategic Studies, infection rates are so high in African armies—20 to 60 percent, depending on the country—that their risk of dying from AIDS is much higher than their risk of combat death.[13] As the United States and Europe rely more on oil from

West Africa, especially from Angola and Nigeria, and are establishing antiter-
rorist command centers in the East African countries of Djibouti, Ethiopia,
Kenya, and Uganda, the HIV/AIDS situation in African armies becomes
more critical to global security. "A key ingredient [in regional security]," says
U.S. Defense Department's Deputy Assistant Secretary for African Affairs,
Theresa Whelan, "is national militaries that are capable and competent and
not dying off because of AIDS."

The U.S. Pentagon spends several million dollars a year helping Angola
and twenty other African countries reduce the risks of HIV in their armies.
But demobilized soldiers in Angola are already infected, carry the virus home
to their villages, and pass it on to wives and girlfriends. Demobilization of
Ethiopian troops after the war with Eritrea spread HIV across the country,
where 10 percent of the adults are now infected. South Africa reports that
one-quarter of its troops are infected. "I wanted to be demobilized," said a
thirty-one-year-old Angolan commando who served in Angola and on UN
peacekeeping missions in three other countries. Looking forward to a normal
life with his wife and children, he was rejected by them when they learned
he was HIV positive. He contemplated suicide. "I fought a lot and I didn't
manage to do almost anything with my life. Now I want to do something
with my life," he protests. "I have children. I have a wife. If I was like other
people who have a lot of money—they go abroad to buy medicines, they go
to South Africa for treatment—then I could continue [my life]."

Sadly, children in Africa and Asia who have lost parents to HIV/AIDS are also
migrating, dropping out of school to look for work in the city or to take care of
sick relatives. According to U.S. Senator Bill Frist, African children growing up
in the shadow of AIDS with little or no guidance from adults constitute "a pool
of recruits for terrorists."[14] Many live in situations of profound abuse with no
parental protection and suffer other losses. "When my father and mother died, I
lived with my uncle," said a child in Malawi. "Then my uncle also got sick and
died, so I went to live with my granny. She could not manage to send me to
school [so I] ended up on the street to work." Sexual abuse and HIV infection of
young children is on the rise in many African countries as more parents die.
According to the South African Law Commission, of the 1.6 million rapes that
occur in South Africa, a country of 42 million people, 20,000 involve children.
"Survival sex" for rent, food, or money is a fact of life for growing numbers of
girls living on the streets and for many working as domestic servants or in mar-
ginally paying jobs. Unprotected vaginal and anal sex is also common among
street boys and girls as a form of initiation, play, or to establish dominance, and
it can be rough. "You don't go halfway," said one street boy in Tanzania, "if you
want to show them what's what."

Other migrants are short-timers or tourists, more like Darwin, curious enough to pursue a one-time encounter with a "beautiful señorita" but too foolish to use protection. Other modern travelers are more predatory—the so-called sex tourists well known in many Asian countries who are interested in more unusual and sometimes pedophiliac sexual encounters that are illegal in their home countries but can be purchased from bribe-paying mafias in well-known tourist destinations. Tourism is an even bigger income generator than migration for work; close to 700 million tourists spent $463.6 billion on jaunts outside their home countries in 2001 according to the World Tourism Organization. The United States is the leading sending and receiving country, grossing $72 billion annually, or 8 percent of the GDP. Tourism, like migration, involves powerful financial incentives for countries as well as for individuals, constituting the first or second largest income producer for many developing countries, especially those in Africa. And high HIV rates are no longer frightening people away. Over the past several years, African tourism has recovered and is increasing dramatically. The Bahamas has a national HIV rate of 3.5 percent, second highest in the Caribbean, but hosts upwards of 3 million tourists each year, more than any other country in the region, because crime rates there are relatively low and facilities are excellent.

The poverty that drives migration is so fundamental that it turns the life of a sufferer into a constant struggle to survive. "Poverty is like living in jail, living under bondage, waiting to be free," says a poor woman in Jamaica.[15] Poverty means loss of freedom, loss of dignity, loss of control over the fundamental course of your life. The poor in Brazil call it "living like a dog," because it makes you so hungry you scavenge, so thirsty you foam at the mouth, so needy you will do anything to make a buck, even sell your body in prostitution. Poverty equates not only with physical suffering and lack of services but with loss of economic and social opportunities and continuous insecurity and anxiety. The poor are denied their rights to services, victimized by public officials, and brutalized by police. Sex is a major part of the economy for poor women, who "form steady, sometimes clandestine, relationships with relatively wealthy men in the hope that it will bring them some material benefit, the occasional chicken perhaps, school fees for the children, or favorable deals for a few cabbages . . . [Sex is] practically the only currency they have."[16] In developing countries without basic social welfare systems, people like Molly, Pauline, and Robina know that their own local institutions and communities are the most reliable source of support.

More than one-quarter of the developing world's people still live in poverty, one-third on incomes of less than $1 a day, and it is in poor countries that HIV/AIDS is the worst. HIV victims in developed countries account for only 4 percent of the global total. Studies in Cambodia, Vietnam, Nicaragua, and Tanzania show that poor people are less likely to know how HIV/AIDS is transmitted or prevented, more likely to have sex at an early age, less likely to use condoms, and more likely, if female, to turn to sex work for support. Studies from Africa, Haiti, and Brazil have demonstrated that poor women are more easily forced into sex work and are less likely to insist on condom use. In Africa, the number of adult women engaging in "survival sex," either full or part time, is high, and their lives often include many episodes of physical abuse and sexual violence.

While Asia has the most people in poverty, the situation is most severe in Africa where the average African household today consumes 20 percent less than it did twenty-five years ago. Sub-Saharan Africa has the largest proportion of people in poverty, 220 million people living without the resources needed to eat a diet sufficient to sustain productive life. In many countries in the subcontinent, close to half of all children and a sizeable minority of adults are malnourished, leaving them highly susceptible to diseases of all types, including HIV/AIDS. The poorest 20 percent of the world's population (4.4 billion people in developing countries) share only 1.1 percent of the world's total income, down from 1.4 percent in 1991 and 2.3 percent in 1960. More than 1 billion are deprived of basic needs, three-fifths lack basic sanitation, one-third are without clean water, one-quarter are without adequate housing, and one-fifth have no access to modern health facilities and schooling. One-fifth of the very poor get too little energy and protein, and 2 billion are anemic.

Poverty and disease are closely interrelated. In developing countries, the most common reason for descent into poverty is the illness, injury, or death of a close family member. When a family member becomes sick with AIDS, the family is rapidly impoverished. They sell their capital goods, land, and livestock, and then their small belongings, and have no cushion if other problems arise. When the food in Ezlina Chambukira's tiny house in Malawi, where 15 percent of the population is infected with HIV, ran out during the 2002 famine, she sold her possessions one by one: a goat, an old umbrella, metal plates, and a battered pail. "I have nothing else to sell," said the thirty-six-year-old woman, drawing her four ragged children close. "I was praying, praying for the rains. I was praying for God to give me food," for the miracle that would save her and her children from sharing the fate of the fourteen people in her village who died from hunger. The climb out of poverty is slow because disposable income is so small and could be lost by chance to natural disasters, poor crops, loss of employment, or another family illness.

�֎ ✷ ✷

A typical Victorian, Darwin admired the South American señoritas but never tells us in his *Journals* or letters what happened next. The fact that he fathered nine children with his wife, Emma, suggests that their use of birth control devices, if any, was not completely effective, although condoms, vaginal diaphragms and caps, and spermicides were widely known in his day. Gabrielle Fallopius first described the condom in 1564 and demonstrated its use for prevention of sexually transmitted diseases in syphilis prevention trials on 1,100 men, who donned linen sheaths, which were sometimes treated with honey, alum, or lactic acid to increase their effectiveness as spermicidal barriers.[17] The condom had been in use for at least 4,000 years before his experiment, depicted on the walls of a 3,000-year-old Egyptian tomb and in early European cave paintings. "Dr. Condom" supplied King Charles II with animal-tissue sheaths to slow his production of illegitimate children and protect him from syphilis. The oldest actual condoms found date from 1640; they were discovered in the foundations of Dudley Castle near Birmingham, England and were made of animal or fish intestines. Gut condoms were scoffed at then as they are now; "real" men claimed they were "an armor against pleasure, a cobweb against infection." Like latex condoms in poorer parts of Africa, the reliability of gut condoms in the seventeenth century may have been compromised by frequent reuse because they were extremely expensive. In 1826 Pope Leo XII banned condoms, believing that the debauched should suffer the consequences of their revels. Public demand did not decline noticeably as a result, and by 1844 Goodyear Rubber was mass-producing condoms from vulcanized rubber. While latex condoms were invented in the 1880s, they did not come into widespread use until the early 1930s. By 1935, 1.5 million condoms were being manufactured each year in the U.S.

The oldest form of birth control is still one of the most effective ways to prevent HIV transmission. When it was first discovered in the mid-1980s that HIV was transmitted in bodily fluids, five ways to prevent HIV transmission were immediately obvious: safe sex through condom use, abstinence, and reduction in the number of sexual partners; testing the blood supply and blood products; and use of clean injecting equipment by drug users. In Eastern Europe and many parts of Asia, the epidemic is spreading out rapidly from core groups of injecting drug users. Moscow alone has 1 million drug users, including 150,000 needle-using cocaine and heroin addicts. Coupled with a flourishing sex trade, where many addicts work, HIV growth is explosive.

In 1994 it was learned that treatment of sexually transmitted diseases (STDs) could reduce HIV transmission by almost half even in the absence of other protective measures because it reduces the amount of virus, or "viral load," present in ejaculations. STDs are strongly correlated with high HIV rates in Africa, where herpes is extremely prevalent in young women shortly after they begin sexual activity. In 1998 it was learned that an inexpensive antiretroviral drug (AZT, or azydothymidine, marketed as Zidovudine or Retrovir) could almost completely block mother-to-child transmission. By 2002 Brazil proved conclusively that antiretroviral treatment not only makes HIV-positive individuals feel better, but reduces their viral load, preventing at last half of the new infections projected for 2002 and turning that nation's epidemic clock back to 1995. Treatment averted 146,000 hospitalizations between 1997 and 1999 because it caused dramatic reductions in opportunistic infections. Best of all, savings realized by the Brazilian government from treatment more than covers the cost of the drugs because Brazil manufacturers its own low-cost antiretrovirals.

Two methods of prevention that can be controlled by women, female condoms and use of microbicides (gels and creams that act as chemical condoms, killing the virus and bacteria that cause sexually transmitted diseases), have never gotten off the ground because they are too expensive or ineffective for widespread use. Feminist protests regarding the failure to find prevention methods that can be controlled by women in an epidemic fueled by their disempowerment have had little effect on international policy. Similarly, debate over male circumcision has been sidestepped since the early 1990s, when Australian demographers Jack and Pat Caldwell and Nigerian demographer I. O. Orubuloye first recognized the coincidence of male circumcision and lower HIV rates, identifying a "non-circumcision belt" traversing the countries of eastern and southern Africa that coincides with high rates of HIV prevalence. HIV infection rates in the Muslim countries of northern Africa and in Muslim populations within highly infected African countries are low, even when they are living side by side and interacting with uncircumcised groups. A UN study of HIV transmission in four African cities found that uncircumcised males were more likely to have AIDS and other curable sexually transmitted diseases. Over forty studies show that uncircumcised men have two to eight times the risk of contracting HIV. The reason is simple: male circumcision fosters improved personal hygiene.

In 1995, while escorting the Caldwells on a week-long tour of HIV/AIDS projects I was managing for the U.S. Agency for International Development (USAID) in Tanzania, the medical director of a tea plantation clinic in the country's remote high central plateau remarked that adult men working on the farm were asking to be circumcised because they heard it helped prevent HIV. The news from Nairobi had reached this farm over hundreds of miles of treacherous African countryside. The Caldwells, who had taken their knocks for having the courage even to mention male circumcision in the international policy arena, felt vindicated: "If the ordinary man is demanding it," Jack remarked, "you know that even if it's 'bad,' it's good!" Despite its effectiveness, adopting male circumcision as a national prevention strategy is still political suicide because only 40 percent of the world's men are circumcised (all Muslims, Jews, Coptic Christians, about three-quarters of all males in the United States and Canada; rates are much lower in Europe).[18] It also runs counter to international condemnation of female circumcision, placing policymakers in a very awkward position.

HIV can be prevented with less radical measures, such as consistent and correct use of a condom, but knowing the biological mechanisms of prevention is only a start. Moving from theory to practice, from small-scale applications to large, creates an entirely different set of problems, although Uganda, Thailand, Cambodia, and Senegal have proven it can be done. By mid-2000 the infection rate in Uganda dropped from 14 percent in the early 1990s to 6.6 percent, and new cases had been halved. Large-scale prevention demands a huge investment of time, money, and commitment by individuals, communities, businesses, and government. Take condom use, the simplest and cheapest form of intervention, as an example. Informing people susceptible to infection how to use a condom and persuading them to do so requires extensive public education, especially for largely illiterate populations with limited media contact. Buying and supplying a sufficient number of condoms and distributing them is costly, especially if road and retail systems are not in place. Even in a thoroughly modernized, relatively rich country like Botswana, with the highest AIDS rate in the world (38.8 percent of the adult population is HIV-positive), the costs are high. If Botswana's 335,000 men each had sex only once a week, they would need 17,422,000 condoms per year, or $871,000 worth of condoms at the wholesale price of $0.05. For poorer countries like Nigeria, with 53 million sexually active adults, or Ethiopia, with 29 million, the costs are astronomical. Of the 8 to 24 billion condoms needed worldwide to prevent HIV, only 6 to 9 billion are distributed annually, and the condom gap in sub-Saharan Africa is at least 2 billion. The cost of closing the gap was $239 million in 2000 and will increase to $557 million by 2015, minus the costs of distribution and education.

Finally, educating governments and other public opinion leaders—especially church officials—that using a condom is necessary or good can be a major stumbling block. When the Catholic church threatened to withdraw its support from his campaign in 1998, former President Frederick Chiluba of Zambia, a country where 20 percent of adults are infected, declared condom advertising illegal. Even prevention of transmission from HIV-positive mothers to infants can become a political football. South Africa has 4.7 million HIV-positive citizens, the largest number in the world, but the government blocked a national prevention program for infants for three years despite the offer of free drugs because the president, Thabo Mbeki, questioned the causal link between HIV and AIDS. In March 2003 South African AIDS activists aligned with the Congress of South African Trade Unions and forced the government to discuss provision of antiretrovirals in the face of a large-scale civil disobedience campaign.

World Bank AIDS expert Martha Ainsworth thinks that governments are reluctant to take responsibility for AIDS prevention because it requires honest talk about sex. "Nearly half of the 4.8 billion people in less-developed countries live in areas where HIV infection is not yet widespread," Ainsworth says, and argues rightly that intelligent action by policymakers could "spare them the ravages of the epidemic." This may be true, but even poor countries committed to providing effective interventions still have to find the money to intervene. Global spending on HIV/AIDS in 2002 was $2.8 billion, less than one-third of the $9.2 billion actually needed. In 2007 prevention will require $15 billion, and by 2015, $25 billion. Of the current total, only $5.4 billion is needed each year in low-income countries (with 96 percent of the cases) because the cost of living is so low. Even so, it is doubtful funding goals will be achieved. Concerted campaigning raised only $2 billion between 2000 and 2002 for the Global AIDS Fund, with slightly more than $600 million dispersed. The United States resists pressure to provide more money to the fund because it removes the political leverage of direct aid and puts decisions about dispersal of the money into the hands of an independent international body of experts. Currently, the United States spends less than half a percent of its GDP on all foreign aid, the lowest of any developed country, and most of it goes to military aid and support for Israel, Egypt, Colombia, and Jordan.

The Global AIDS Fund, an independent public-private partnership, has received huge private contributions but measly public support. Bill and Melinda Gates gave $100 million on the first round compared to $250 million from the U.S. government. Developed countries are asked to give .035 percent of their GDP, so the United States should provide 44 percent of the Fund's capital. By 2003, it had pledged $1.65 billion, nearly half of the fund's total pledges. That was increased to $5 billion over five years in May 2003, but only if the U.S. contribution amounts to no more than one-third of the fund's total. The Netherlands, Sweden, and Italy have fulfilled the

request, but Japan met only 12 percent of the requested amount, and other
wealthy countries have followed suit. Much of the $15 billion the United
States committed to spend in 2003 on AIDS, a small fraction of the cost of
mobilization for the war in Iraq, is drawn out of current programs in child
health. Lobbyists for increased funding even include the African Wildlife
Foundation, the United State's oldest African conservation group, which is
worried that the economic and social havoc created by the epidemic in Africa
is causing wholesale "destructive uses of land, water, and natural resources"
and that "the ecological toll will never be recovered or reversed."

Poor countries devote huge portions of their budget to debt service and
have little left over to invest even in basic healthcare. Africa spent $14 billion
in 2002 alone on debt service, considerably more than it needs to prevent
HIV/AIDS. The outstanding debt of the thirty-three of the world's thirty-
eight "highly indebted countries" (HIPC) in Africa averages four times
annual export earnings, effectively undermining all social spending. The
reluctance to forgive African debt can be contrasted with the situation in
1953, when the United States wrote off half of Germany's debt and resched-
uled the remaining half so it would consume less than 5 percent of the country's annual export income. In 1998 President Bill Clinton canceled the debt
African countries owed the U.S. government, but countries struggle with
repayment of their International Monetary Fund (IMF) and World Bank
borrowings. Since 2000 only six countries have been able to swing agreements with the IMF and World Bank to swap "debt for AIDS"—commit
their savings from debt forgiveness to HIV prevention and care. At their
April 2002 board meetings, the IMF and World Bank announced they
were tightening the screws on five of these countries, a move that outraged
Britain's treasury chief Gordon Brown so much that he asked the UN
General Assembly in May for an additional $1 billion in debt relief to "ensure
a robust exit from unsustainable debt." He urged wealthy countries to channel an additional $50 billion each year into help for developing countries, an
effort he called a "global Marshall Plan."

AIDS activists are demanding that transnational corporations provide
HIV/AIDS prevention and care for their employees. Twenty-nine of the
world's top one hundred economic entities are companies, and their value
has grown faster than countries over the past ten years. Exxon, for example,
is comparable to Chile or Pakistan in value, Nigeria ranks between
DaimlerChrysler and General Electric, and Phillip Morris exceeds Tunisia,
Slovakia, and Guatemala. Many companies in Africa, such as British
American Tobacco, DeBeers Diamonds, and Anglo American Mines (which
estimates that 20 percent of its workforce in forty countries is HIV positive),

began providing prevention, diagnosis, and treatment for African workers after studies showed how high their replacement costs would be for deaths from AIDS. Coca-Cola, one of the largest private sector employers in Africa, was providing full medical coverage for 1,500 direct employees and family members and free advertising space and marketing know-how for HIV prevention, but activists wanted more. After fifteen months of badgering through international e-mail campaigns and live protests, Coke, which made $630 million from cola sales in Africa in 2001, agreed to provide care for another 98,500 workers who are bottlers, canners, and distributors under contract arrangement with the company.

Finally, poor countries are still fighting the pharmaceutical industry, backed by the World Trade Organization (WTO) and the U.S. government, for the right to manufacture or purchase low-cost AIDS drugs.[19] In 2000 the United States allied itself with the pharmaceutical industry to threaten economic sanctions against Brazil, South Africa, Zimbabwe, and other countries using cheap imported or home-made generic versions of anti-AIDS drugs to reduce treatment costs for an individual from $10,000 per year to $300. After a media and e-mail campaign led by Médecins Sans Frontieres (Doctors Without Borders), public indignation was so intense that pharmaceutical giants dropped their lawsuits. In 2001 the UN Commission on Human Rights declared that access to medicine was an essential human right and asked member states to "refrain from taking measures which would deny or limit equal access" to HIV/AIDS drugs and actively "facilitate access" of poor countries to drugs, including their manufacture. Drug factories in Kenya and other African countries are producing generic AIDS medicines, anticipating a successful legal challenge to WTO prohibitions. African drug companies have made generic copies of many different drugs for decades, paying royalties to western drug companies with patented formulas. In March 2002, the World Health Organization (WHO) included generic AIDS drugs on its approved list and the European Union and United Nations Children's Fund (UNICEF) agreed to finance generics, but big drug companies still refuse to accept the idea that they should not be the only ones making life-or-death decisions about access to these drugs. Brazil, intimidated by the United States and the WTO, refused to sell its generic AIDS drugs to other Latin American countries. When a thirty-six-year-old Honduran mother of four died in 2002 because she could not afford drugs, the Pan American Health Organization stepped in to negotiate an average 55 percent price reduction from five brand name manufacturers and even better deals from generic producers.

AIDS activists have accused drug makers collaborating with UNAIDS in "Accelerating Access," an initiative to furnish drugs to more people with

HIV/AIDS in developing countries, of "profiting from a partnership with international institutions while using the program to keep their monopolies and to limit any reductions in price." In two years the program furnished drugs to less than 0.1 percent of the people who needed them. In the meantime, pharmaceutical companies remained the most profitable sector of the U.S. economy for the third decade, ranking at the top of all of *Fortune Magazine*'s measures of profitability, prompting Frank Clemente of Public Citizen's Congress Watch to remark that "during a year in which there was much talk of sacrifice in the national interest, drug companies increased their astounding profits" by 32 percent in 2001 when other industries declined by 53 percent. Clemente attributed this to "advertising some medicines more than Nike shoes" and lobbying campaigns that keep U.S. congressmen safely in drug company pockets, extending "lucrative monopoly patents. Sometimes what's best for shareholders and chief executive officers isn't what's best for all Americans, particularly senior citizens who lack insurance coverage for prescription drugs." In early 2003 Swiss drug maker Roche announced a new AIDS drug with a record-breaking price of $20,000 per year, more than double the cost of any other drug on the market, which the firm concedes will definitely put it out of the reach of anyone in developing countries.

"In the end," says International AIDS Vaccine Initiative director Seth Berkley, who cut his teeth as an epidemiologist in Brazil and Uganda in the 1980s, "only a vaccine will matter" because "we are still fooling around on the edges" of prevention. Two things work against making a vaccine a reality: insufficient investment, which Berkley tries to address through the Vaccine Initiative, and scientific ability to apply knowledge of molecular genetics to the problem. At least thirty other AIDS vaccines are in various stages of development, but the virus' ability to hide in white blood cells eludes standard vaccine technology. VaxGen, the California company farthest ahead in the vaccine race, reported relatively high success in blacks and Asians from its first clinical trials in February 2003, but the vaccine was virtually ineffective in whites and Hispanics. Most experts agree with National Institute of Health physician Anthony Fauci, who believes "it will eventually happen. But there are many problems we need to solve in order to produce one. I would have to say the virus is winning, not us."

✹ ✹ ✹

On the tenth World AIDS Day, December 1, 1997, experts from UNAIDS, the combined UN agency leading the global AIDS fight, revealed they had been significantly underestimating HIV and AIDS worldwide. This bias had existed for at least five years according to their director, Dr. Peter Piot. Official AIDS estimates still understate the actual numbers by one-quarter to one-third. One reason, it seems, is to avoid panic, not to mention the embarrassment that comes with being wrong. In the mid-1980s, the world's first AIDS modelers had their ears pinned back when they predicted a much more vigorous epidemic in England than actually occurred. Politicians control the availability of data from many countries, and more than a few careers have been broken by bad statistics. In the 1990s many African countries deliberately minimized their HIV/AIDS data out of fear that overly adverse reports would deter millions of tourists and international business investment. Businesses do not want to be stuck with losses from high health and death benefits or the constant hassle of recruiting and training replacement workers.

The major reason for underestimation, however, is that HIV/AIDS numbers are so difficult to interpret and project. The spread of HIV infection far outdistances any means of detecting it in the early years of a country's epidemic, and surges can be delayed for years or hidden within national averages. HIV showed up in Thailand in 1984 but did not spread aggressively among sex workers and their clients for five years. In Nepal, HIV infections among needle-sharing drug users grew slowly for seven years, until by 1997 more than half were HIV positive. Growth can be sudden, jumping from 4 to 61 percent among sex workers in Nairobi, Kenya between 1981 and 1985, or start more slowly, increasing from 0 to 2 percent in Nairobi's pregnant women from 1981 to 1985, and then enter a sharp rise. For most diseases, actual cases are usually ten to one hundred times more common than reported cases because people have no symptoms or seek no care.[20] Even in the United States, where reporting AIDS is mandatory and care is provided, a study in South Carolina showed that 40 percent of AIDS cases had gone unreported.

The gap between countries' reported HIV/AIDS cases and HIV prevalence (the actual cases in the population) can be very significant. For example, Vietnam now has several thousand AIDS cases, but experts estimate that at least 150,000 Vietnamese are HIV positive. The former figure, along with outdated prevalence data, were reported to UNAIDS for aggregation into the 2002 international report, so the global estimate for Vietnam is off by at least a factor of ten. In 1999, 32.6 percent of the women coming to Swaziland's prenatal clinics were HIV-positive, but the country reported virtually no cases to UNAIDS. India, Russia, and China are all underreporting and are unable or unwilling to monitor their respective epidemics closely or devise national responses adequate to confront the wave of devastation and death that is coming.

International HIV/AIDS statistics are prepared by UNAIDS, a seven-year-old coalition of eight United Nations agencies[21] established in 1996 after a bloody four-year battle for control within the UN "family." WHO traditionally takes leadership on international disease issues, but the multisectoral nature of HIV/AIDS—the fact that it can be managed only if the health sector collaborates with other sectors—led other UN agencies to seek equal roles. Each UN group recognized that the agency chosen to lead the global fight against AIDS could leverage millions of dollars in funding at a time when budgets from other sources were running thin. Piot, a personable and experienced Belgian tropical medicine hero who made his name fighting the Ebola virus in the Congo, helped divide up the turf and has led this "peer among equals agency" ever since. To avoid renewing the conflict, the Global Fund for AIDS, Tuberculosis and Malaria was created as an independent foundation in 2000.

Many people living with HIV/AIDS "go underground" because of stigma or ignorance, and many deaths are falsely attributed to tuberculosis, pneumonia, or other opportunistic infections. Families do not want the true cause of a loved one's death known, and even if they did, there are not enough HIV test kits to confirm diagnoses in developing countries. The poverty of health-care systems leaves 90 percent of those who are HIV-positive unaware of their status and 40 to 50 percent of AIDS sufferers without medical attention of any kind. Internationally, less than 4 percent of HIV-positive people in poor countries have access to antiretroviral treatments and less than 10 percent have access to treatment for opportunistic infections (tuberculosis, skin problems, diarrhea) or pain medication of any kind. Tony Moll, head of a 350-bed hospital in South Africa says, "we have no medicines for AIDS. So many hospitals tell [AIDS victims] 'You've got AIDS. We can't help you. Go home and die.'" Moll says that no one volunteers for an HIV test because "if the choice is to know and get nothing, they don't want to know."

From the microbe's perspective, genetics is not a rigid blueprint but more like a game of Scrabble, where each organism internally manipulates its letters, passing some on to its neighbors while trying to hide what it's doing from opponents.[22] Viruses are alive but will not stay that way for long without help because they cannot "eat" or reproduce by themselves. They manipulate host cells in bacteria, animals, and humans to survive but do not cause cell death, tissue injury, or illness unless an environmental change initiates a different response. HIV, a retrovirus, is unlike most other viruses and all other cellular organisms because it carries its genetic information in RNA (ribonucleic acid) instead of DNA (deoxyribonucleic acid). Using a special reverse transcriptase enzyme, it reverses its host cell's normal process of changing DNA into RNA to make the DNA it needs to reproduce. Other retroviruses cause liver cancer and leukemia in humans.

Human immunodeficiency virus, or HIV, belongs to a subset of retroviruses called lentiviruses that cause slow progressive diseases. Its closest relative, SIV or simian immunodeficiency virus, is found in *Pan troglodytes troglodytes*, a chimp in equatorial West Africa. HIV has crossed the species barrier more than once, most recently about seventy years ago. Other members of the HIV family are found in cows, sheep, horses, and cats, which have lived with the virus for a longer time and are immune to debilitating infection. One of the common misperceptions about HIV is that it passed from monkeys to humans through sex. While HIV did jump from monkeys to humans, it made the leap because Africans eat "bush meat," hunting monkeys and other wild animals for food in the same way that Americans hunt deer, squirrel, snakes, and even capture frogs to eat, an idea Africans find abhorrent. In 2002 researchers screening blood from 573 monkeys sold as meat and 215 kept as pets in Cameroon found that a fifth tested positive for HIV and its relatives. Other related viruses have also crossed into humans but have not caused epidemics. Most cross-species transmissions go nowhere, according to Beatrice Hahn, one of the University of Alabama researchers involved in the study.

HIV was discovered in 1983 at a time when only two other retroviruses had been identified, both by Robert Gallo of the National Institutes of Health (NIH) in Bethesda, Maryland. Just as scientific investigation into evolution was occurring simultaneously in several places during Darwin's time, HIV was identified as the cause of AIDS by Gallo and three other groups of scientists in 1983–1984: Luc Montagnier of the Pasteur Institute in Paris, Jay Levy at the University of California/San Francisco, and a group of Centers for Disease Control (CDC) researchers. Gallo first cultivated the virus in a lab so that a diagnostic test could be developed in 1985. Lacking Darwin and Wallace's amiability, the relationship between Pasteur Institute and NIH scientists was strained by a press and public eager to know which one had actually "discovered" the virus. Their governments mediated, giving both equal credit and allocating the test kit royalties to a foundation to fight HIV/AIDS in African countries, which already had the worst epidemics in the world.

A single HIV particle looks like a rubber ball covered with suction cups that help the virus stick to its host cells through chemical interaction. Thousands of times smaller than the cells they infect, 250,000 HIV particles laid end to end barely make an inch. Like the organisms in Darwin's shipboard dust, HIV has enormous adaptive ability but is extremely fragile outside of the human body. Compared to cold viruses, for instance, that can linger on for days on doorknobs and other surfaces, HIV dies within hours when it hits the air, is rendered inactive by bleach, alcohol, or soap and water, and is vulnerable to the stomach acids that protect us from a whole array of other germs. HIV is virulent and crafty when inside the body. Sneaking into cell nuclei and cloning itself, it mutates rapidly to avoid recognition by the immune system and reproduces on a massive scale. When an HIV-positive person gets a disease like tuberculosis or pneumonia, HIV overwhelms the immune system and the patient dies.

There are three main strains of HIV, and eleven subtypes identified by a letter from A to K. When HIV first appeared, different subtypes were clearly associated with the major modes of transmission, but since HIV mutates freely, new combinations of the basic subtypes can occur. When HIV was first identified in China, for example, the predominant form of the virus was subtype E, brought into coastal settlements by visiting sailors. Subtype C arrived from India, then B showed up among injecting drug users. C and B recombined and are moving rapidly northward and into the interior. New combinations develop within individuals who acquire two types. A drug user, for example, can get the B subtype from sharing needles and C from a sexual contact. During vaccine trials in Thailand, the dominant subtype, B, was almost completely replaced by subtype E in the test group in only a few years.

� ✗ ✗

As was true with the worldwide syphilis epidemic that began in the sixteenth century, one of the major causes for the rapid spread of AIDS is ignorance. A 2002 UNAIDS survey in three dozen countries found that even where infection rates were high, two-thirds of women and 80 percent of men said they were either at no risk or low risk for AIDS. In countries where 20 to 30 percent of the population is HIV positive, this idea is at best naively optimistic. Half the respondents to 2000 and 2002 surveys in 28 countries say they are unconcerned about getting STDs and 38 percent take no measures to protect themselves.[23] Indian AIDS expert Siddhartha Dube argues that the detailed information sexually active people need to protect themselves is usually not provided by prevention campaigns. General slogans like "Love

Carefully" do not give anyone the explicit information they need to protect themselves.

Since women are much less well informed than men, the virus is spreading much more rapidly among females everywhere. Globally, 54 percent of all HIV-positive people are female; in Africa it's two-thirds. Up to one-quarter of women in countries with low HIV rates like Jordan, and high rates like Mozambique, do not know that AIDS is fatal. Even if women are aware, their right to refuse sex is limited. In India as in Africa, men who have sex outside of marriage experience no stigma, but if their wives demand condom use, they risk partner violence. Almost half of all women in Ethiopia, Uganda, and Kenya, a third in Canada, and a fifth in the United States have been beaten by their husbands, the most common form of violence against women in every country. The CDC estimates that the health-related costs of rape, physical assault, stalking, and homicide by intimate partners exceeds $5.8 billion each year in the United States alone. The ultimate costs are even higher because many women and children do not seek medical assistance. According to U.S. Health and Human Services Secretary Tommy Thompson, "violence against women harms more than its direct victim. It also harms the children, the abuser, and the entire health of all our families and communities."

In Africa many women believe they deserve a beating (as long as it does not leave visible marks) if dinner is not ready on time or if they go out without their husband's permission, and men agree. Women with HIV are much more likely to have a physically violent partner, and almost half said they could not deny their husbands sex after a beating or if they feared HIV infection. Women have more illnesses but are less likely to receive medical treatment, and girls, not boys, are taken out of school to replace lost labor from AIDS deaths in families or to care for sick family members. In Swaziland, school enrollment has fallen more than a third due to AIDS, and most of the students withdrawn were girls. The loss is everyone's. A World Bank study in sub-Saharan Africa showed that gender discrimination has reduced per capita economic growth in the region by 0.8 percent each year since 1960, roughly the same annual loss experts attribute to AIDS. Almost 70 percent of the world's 1.2 billion extremely poor people are women.

HIV/AIDS epidemics vary widely between neighboring countries and within national borders, and also change over time. When HIV first hit the United States, its victims were members of what was sardonically called the "4-H club": homosexuals, heroin users, Haitians, and hemophiliacs. Largely because of its aggressive "migration" into minority populations through bisexuals and injecting drug users, it was the top killer of men and women ages eighteen to thirty-four and now infects almost as many women as men. Aggressive treatment for AIDS has cut deaths from HIV in the United States by 70 percent since 1994, but it is still the sixth leading cause of death between ages twenty-five and forty-four, hitting blacks and Hispanics in this age group disproportionately. New infections can increase rapidly and unexpectedly. A new drug, crystal meth (amphetamine), or "crystal dick" as it is known in the gay community, makes the user "ravenously horny" and is linked to an upsurge of high risk sexual behavior and HIV among young homosexuals. Incidence among injecting drug users is declining because of needle exchange programs, and in 2002 only 20 percent of New York City's injecting drug users were positive compared to more than half in 1990. New York has 50,000 cases of AIDS among injecting drug users, their partners, and their children, more than the total in many European countries and some countries in Africa. Over the past few years, AIDS has also migrated into rural populations in the Southern United States, where seven of the states with the top ten AIDS case rates are located.

More than half of all U.S. adults do not know if they are HIV positive. Although it is easy to get a free HIV test, 41 percent of people diagnosed with AIDS did not get tested until they fell sick, either at the same time as their AIDS diagnosis or within the year before it, giving them more than seven years to infect their partners. While 60 percent of Americans polled in 2000 said they are concerned about contracting sexually transmitted diseases, 30 percent take no protective measures. Most said they still blame people with HIV/AIDS for getting it, but do not know how the disease is actually transmitted, although Americans have sex more often and have a higher number of lifetime partners than any other developed country (124 times per year, a lifetime average of 14.3 partners). Japanese respondents reported an average of 37 times a year, the lowest of any country surveyed.

Young Americans are having sex at increasingly younger ages and have more partners by the time they reach twenty than their parents dreamed of in a lifetime. The average sixteen- to twenty-year-old has already had five partners, gaining ground quickly on twenty-five- to thirty-four-year-olds with eight partners and those over forty-five who report an average of nine. The University of Minnesota's Center for Adolescent Health and Development reports that 34 percent of ninth graders in the United States have had sexual intercourse. A seventeen-year old who has had seven partners says that pregnancy is a more immediate concern than HIV, although "the anxiety [about AIDS] never leaves me. But I still have sex. And I know I can always get oral sex without getting too emotionally involved." Only African teens have sex more often than Americans. At least one-third of young African women are married by eighteen, and half have had sex. Of these, half want to use birth control but cannot get it, so the rate of unintended pregnancy is 20 percent. Like teens in the United States, over half of the Africans do not think they are at risk for AIDS.

These trends are part of a worldwide pattern. More than one-third of African girls and boys surveyed had given or received gifts or money in exchange for sex. Japan's *puchi-iede*, schoolgirls who use their cell phones to hook up with men twice their age for "compensated dating," trade pictures of prospective customers through high tech video displays. Since most young women in almost every culture have their first sexual experience with an older male, far more young women than young men are infected in most countries. In Africa, females between ages fifteen and nineteen are five or six times more likely to be infected than men in the same age group. The dynamic for many is the one that Molly and Pauline discussed in Rakai, with older men enticing younger girls into sex by offering them desperately needed money or promises of favors like good grades on their school exams.

The age of puberty has dropped continuously since 1900 due to improved nutrition, so some of the explanation for the rapid increase in teen sex may be physical. But for teenagers, sex is more than a way to satisfy raging hormones. It is part of broader exploration of the world and a way to separate from their families and form new social bonds that may require rebellious and even destructive or copycat behavior, like injecting drug use or suicide, a common cause of death among young people worldwide. Many of their coming-of-age behaviors put them at risk of HIV infection. More than 5 million U.S. teens, 23 percent in a 2002 survey, said they had unprotected sex because of alcohol or drug abuse, cross-over behavior that contributes to rapid HIV spread. The National Survey of Family Growth, which interviewed 1,280 teen girls between fifteen and nineteen, found that adolescents using birth control were no more sexually active than nonusers and were more likely to use protection when they had sex. Government programs had little effect, but the quality of family and community life is critical in shaping young people's behavior.

In the few African countries with epidemic decline or slowdown, the most important factor is a change in teen sexual norms. In the late 1980s, young Ugandans began delaying their first sexual experience because of AIDS, so the proportion that had intercourse before their twenties was halved by 1995. Change in teen norms is vital to stop HIV spread because the majority of new infections occur among young people. By the end of 1998, one-third of all HIV-positive or AIDS-infected people around the world were between ages fifteen and twenty-four, and more than half of all new infections are within that age group. Six young people are infected with HIV every minute, resulting in 8,500 new infections every day. More than 10 million fifteen- to twenty-four-year-olds are now living with HIV and will develop AIDS during the next three to fifteen years.

HIV infection in teens will continue to define the epidemic and global population structure for the next three decades. Between 1960 and 1990, when HIV/AIDS took hold, the proportion of young people in the world doubled; today more than half of the world's population is under twenty-five. By 2025, the average age will increase only five years to thirty. The world is young and will not get much older until the middle of this century, especially the developing world, where 85 percent of young people live and where close to 95 percent of persons living with HIV/AIDS are concentrated. High infection rates among young people mean that epidemic's global drag will be even greater. Young people get sick just when they reach their prime productive years, wasting their society's investment in education and job training. They also live longer and need more care than older people with the virus. The United Nations Development Program claims that "never before in history have death rates of this magnitude been seen among young adults of both sexes and from all walks of life."

Young people are not alone in taking sexual risks. AIDS has thrown the window on human sexual behavior wide open. Since the early 1980s, experience in country after country has shown that scientists and politicians who thought that infection could be confined to "high risk" groups (sex workers, homosexuals, injecting drug users, soldiers) were wrong. As AIDS epidemics have become increasingly heterosexual everywhere, scientists learned that "ordinary" people network with "high risk" individuals, who also interact with one another. Many homosexual and bisexual men have sex with wives and other female partners in Latin America, Asia, and the Middle East. African men and women were thought to be exclusively heterosexual, but same sex behavior has been documented among men confined in mining camps or prisons. Anal sex is a common heterosexual practice in many cultures, and pedophilia is more common than was believed. A significant minority of men and women around the world engage in bestiality, or sex with animals. In 1948 sex researcher Alfred Kinsey found that 8 percent of American males and 3.6 percent of females had had sex with animals sometime in their lives, including half of all men living in rural areas. In the 1970s the overall proportion had dropped to 5 percent as more farms disappeared, but proponents claim that interest is again on the rise in urban populations.[24] "The presumption that most people are heterosexual and the idea that heterosexuality and homosexuality represent sharply distinct behaviors seem reasonable to most of us. But human behavior is far more complex than that," says human sexuality expert Anne Fausto-Sterling.

�֍ ✖ ✖

Seventy percent of all HIV-positive people in the world today live in sub-Saharan Africa, where 9 percent of the overall population is infected (compared to 0.6 percent of adults in the United States). Of the world's total 28 million AIDS deaths to date, 26 million have been in sub-Saharan Africa. By 2010 at least 18 million additional Africans will die, but the new death toll could easily top 30 million if infection rates in Nigeria and Ethiopia become as high as predicted. More than 15 percent of the subcontinent's population will have died of AIDS by 2010, and another 5 percent (60 to 85 million people) will be living with the infection. In the Arab countries of northern Africa (Morocco, Western Sahara, Mauritania, Algeria, Tunisia, Libya, and Egypt), only 0.1 percent of adults are infected, with the exception of Sudan at 2.5 percent. Botswana, in southern Africa, has the world's highest national rate: 38.8 percent. One-third of adults in the countries of Lesotho, Swaziland, and Zimbabwe are HIV-positive, as are one-fifth of Namibia and Zambia's adults, 15 percent of Kenya's adults, and 5 to 10 percent of adults in most other sub-Saharan countries. HIV surveys in South Africa in 2002 suggest that HIV infection may be leveling off at 25 percent of the population with 4.74 million infected. A handful of countries outside of Africa have higher rates, including several countries in the Caribbean, Latin America, and Asia, but only Haiti, at 6 percent, has an epidemic anywhere near as severe as sub-Saharan Africa.

The impact of the HIV/AIDS epidemic in sub-Saharan Africa will be measured in decades, not in years. Infection levels in Africa will stay high through at least 2010 and the number of deaths will increase over the next twenty years because of the lag between infection and death. Adult death rates had already doubled in the 1990s, and the combined burden of early death and debilitation became four times higher than in the western world. Tuberculosis increased as much as five times over preepidemic levels from interaction with HIV, and resistant strains make tuberculosis much harder to control. Karen Stanecki, chief of the Health Studies Branch at the U.S. Bureau of Census, says that the AIDS pandemic is dramatically changing the demographic makeup of African countries. By 2010, five countries will have negative population growth and eleven will have life expectancies of only thirty years, a statistic not seen since the end of the 1800s.

One of the most tragic measures of epidemic impact in sub-Saharan Africa is the huge and growing number of orphans in the region. In 2001, 11 million African children under fifteen were orphaned by AIDS. When added to the 23 million whose parents died of other causes, there were more than 34 million children, 12 percent of all children under fifteen, who had lost one or both parents. By 2005 that total will be 39 million, and by 2010, 42 million. These estimates were made before the startling epidemic takeoff in Nigeria and Ethiopia, so by the end of the decade, the number of orphans is likely to be two to three times official estimates. Without AIDS, the number of orphans in the region would have declined by 2010.

All of these statistics speak of massive pressure on existing social systems that will continue for decades. Teachers are dying faster than they can be trained. One-fifth of all college students in South Africa's Kwa Zulu Natal Province are HIV positive. AIDS, malaria, and tuberculosis have overwhelmed their healthcare systems. In heavily infected countries, upward of 50 percent of hospital beds are occupied by AIDS patients, increasing deaths among HIV-negative patients who cannot get care. Public health spending is consumed by AIDS to the detriment of childhood vaccination programs and other routine care. In 1999 a WHO study of home care for AIDS patients in Botswana found that most did not have enough food to eat, a common condition in neighboring countries as well. AIDS deaths in the ten hardest hit African countries is reducing the rural labor force by as much as 26 percent, badly cutting into subsistence food production. "Throughout history," the UN Food and Agriculture Organization (FAO) concluded, "few crises have presented such a threat to human health and social and economic progress as does the HIV/AIDS pandemic." In 2002 it warned that vast amounts of humanitarian aid will soon be needed to avert mass starvation in many African countries.

The UN's International Labour Office (ILO) estimates that the labor force will be 20 percent smaller by 2010 because of premature loss of experienced workers to AIDS. "The epidemic affects social and economic life in ways we have never seen before," says ILO's AIDS director, Franklyn Lisk. "The main socio-economic impact of HIV/AIDS is its decimation of the labour force and the level and allocation of savings and investment. This portends a huge humanitarian disaster with dire economic and social consequences. Decades of gains in development, training, skills and education are being lost forever," he said. The UN Development Program predicts increases in crime and, with widening disparities between income groups, breakdown of social order.

Without much more help from the outside, the epidemic in sub-Saharan Africa is unlikely to slow or stabilize over the next decade or two, and social and economic conditions will not stabilize for at least two decades after that.

✻ ✻ ✻

Twenty years ago, when AIDS was first discovered in sub-Saharan Africa, the very immune systems of the communities where it took hold had already been devastated. The basic requisites for decent human existence—food, clothing, water, sanitation, shelter, employment, access to healthcare and education—were beyond the reach of most people. Individual immune systems had been weakened by relentless malnutrition and by curable STDs and other illnesses, rampant because of lack of water, sanitation, and medical treatment. There was no residual strength left to fight AIDS when it came. Experts blame the structural adjustment policies of international development banks for Africa's relentless decline since the 1980s. According to Salih Booker of the Washington-based advocacy group, Foreign Policy in Focus, "the IMF and the World Bank have much to answer for. [Their] policies have eroded Africa's health care systems and intensified the poverty of Africa's people. These institutions must be made accountable for their role in causing the worst health crisis in human history, which Africa now faces."

AIDS took off in Africa before the HIV virus had been identified and linked to it, before there were any tests to detect HIV, before epidemic tracking systems existed, and before antiretroviral treatments were discovered. While HIV/AIDS was building steam in sub-Saharan Africa, scientific understanding of how to prevent the disease was limited. As the epidemic worsened, arguments about the best approach to take caused long program delays. Once prevention programs started, the breakdown of African infrastructure, illiteracy, and widespread poverty meant that few services were available and that ways to communicate about the disease were limited. African politicians and scientists had a fatal skepticism about the disease, suspecting it had been created by white men to scare Africans into population control. Some even thought that the disease had been created by the U.S. Central Intelligence Agency.

These fears were very real for African policymakers who had experienced excessive abuse and exploitation during colonial and postcolonial periods. The wholesale rape of Africa had been going on for many centuries before the World Bank was created in 1945. The continual hardships and lost opportunities experienced by Pauline, Molly, and Robina are not unique in Africa and are a direct outcome of exploitation by European and American slavers, colonialists, and strategists who viewed the continent as a private preserve from the early seventeenth century until African independence in the 1960s. From the perspective of history, AIDS is only the latest of the many tragedies that have scarred the subcontinent since the 1600s.

CHAPTER THREE

Africa's Political and Economic Development

"Wherever the European has trod," Darwin told his Victorian audience at the close of his *Journals*, "death seems to pursue the aboriginal. We may look to the wide extent of the Americas, Polynesia, the Cape of Good Hope, and Australia, and we find the same result. Nor is it the white man alone that thus acts the destroyer," he continued. "The Polynesian of Malay extraction has in parts of the East Indian archipelago, thus driven before him the dark coloured-native. The varieties of man," he mused, "seem to act on each other in the same way as different species of animals—the stronger always extirpating the weaker." Darwin had already seen the fate of Jeremy Button and the Tierra del Fuegians, and the terrible effects of slavery on Africans and their descendents in Brazil.

After only two months aboard, Darwin nearly abandoned the *Beagle* following a disagreement with Fitz Roy about slavery. He had turned a blind eye to Fitz Roy's cruelty when he brutally flogged two crew members for getting drunk on Christmas Day, but when the captain declared that slaves were better off under their owner's care than dying in poverty as free men, Darwin could not hold his tongue. His grandfathers and their Quaker friends had started the British antislavery movement in 1780, forcing Parliament to ban the slave trade in all British dominions in 1807. By 1828, a year before Darwin left on the *Beagle*, free people of color were put on the same legal footing as whites in British colonies. As Britain pulled out of the slave trade, the French, Portuguese, and Spanish took up the slack. In 1832, as Parliament began debate on a bill requiring full emancipation in its colonies, Darwin was getting firsthand experience of what the institution of slavery in Brazil was all about.

Slavery had been big business in the country for 150 years when Darwin landed there in 1831, and it continued until 1850, when Britain threatened to seize the slavers' ships. Darwin found Brazil a "scandal to Christian nations" because half the population was in slavery. "I thank God I shall never again visit a slave-country . . . I heard the most pitiable moans, and could not but suspect that some poor slave was being tortured, yet knew I was powerless as a child even to remonstrate," he cried. In Bahía, Darwin lived opposite an old Spanish woman who crushed her female slaves' fingers with thumbscrews, and knew that Brazilian slave hunters sliced the ears off their captives. "I have stayed in a house where a young household mulatto, daily and hourly, was reviled, beaten, and persecuted enough to break the spirit of the lowest animal," he wrote. "I have seen a little boy, six or seven years old, struck thrice with a horse whip (before I could interfere) on his naked head, for having handed me a glass of water not quite clean."

Darwin urged his readers to "picture to yourself the chance, ever hanging over you, of your wife and your little children . . . torn from you and sold like beasts to the first bidder!" He told them how the brutality of slavery could damage the human dignity of the master as well as the slave. "I was crossing a ferry with a negro," he wrote, and "in endeavoring to make him understand, I talked loud, and made signs . . . passed my hand near his face. He . . . thought I was in a passion, and was going to strike him; for instantly, with a frightened look and half-shut eyes, he dropped his hands. I shall never forget my feelings of surprise, disgust, and shame, at seeing a great powerful man afraid even to ward off a blow, directed, as he thought, at his face. This man had been trained to a degradation lower than . . . the most helpless animal. These deeds are done," Darwin said, "by men who profess to love their neighbor as themselves, who believe in God, and pray that his Will be done on earth! It makes one's blood boil, yet heart tremble," he continued, "to think that we Englishmen and our American descendents, with their boastful cry of liberty, have been and are so guilty."

�֍ ✖ ✖

"Sex with monkeys?" Molly exclaimed, incredulous, and looked nervously around the room to see if anyone else had heard Pauline. "They think we have sex with monkeys," Pauline repeated, even louder than before, and several heads turned to eavesdrop on the rangy woman, slumped over her second cup of tea. Rakai's Little Blue Room Restaurant chapattis were the best in the county, especially when they were served with a cup of tea made with fresh milk from a long-horned Ankole cow. Molly had helped Josephine

Rutayaga hang the tiny white Christmas lights along the blue painted tree branch that arched across the middle of the small room, optically separating the front from the back. Even so, the room was only large enough to fit two small tables, one on either side of the twig divide, so it was hard to get any privacy in the tiny restaurant. The Blue had been a favorite of the Tanzanian soldiers, who celebrated their victory over Amin's army there with a wild party.

Born before independence in 1954, Molly was the third daughter of a teacher at the colony's proudest secondary school. When Idi Amin took the reins of power and began slowly killing Uganda's intellectuals to dumb down the resistance, her father had fled to Kenya. Molly had followed him with her mother, brother, and sisters, slipping across the border at night to avoid Amin's drunken guards. The family had settled in the Lake Victoria town of Kisumu, where her father taught school and her brother worked as a fisherman. As soon as the Tanzanians deposed Amin, Molly's father moved the family back to Uganda, but decided to settle far away from Kampala's incendiary politics of revenge. So they came to Rakai district, famous over the next decade for two things: It was the first Uganda district in the path of the triumphal march of Julius Nyerere's army that liberated Uganda from Amin, and it was, not unrelatedly, thought to be the birthplace of AIDS.

Thanks to Uganda's forgiving soil, most people in the countryside were able to ride out the economic breakdown resulting from Amin's arbitrary terrorism. In Rakai district, coping took two other forms: for men, black market smuggling, bringing goods across Lake Victoria from Tanzania, and for women, prostitution. Dishonesty was a prerequisite for survival, values were turned upside down, and morals collapsed along with the economy. Uganda's new president, Yowero Museveni, faced a double challenge, Molly thought, moral as well as economic reconstruction.

"Your face is so sunburned," Pauline said, "what have you been up to?" "I've been helping Mrs. Kasadha plant her new garden," Molly replied. "That woman in Kansansero living with her twelve grandchildren?" "That's the one," Molly said. "Her daughter died, leaving her with the first six, then her son in Mkono passed away. His wife was already dead, so she got their six too. I think AIDS is going to kill the old lady by starving her and those kids out. There's no place to send them. None of the other relatives will help, but the old lady wants to keep them all. She told an aid worker the other day that if they'd just give her the money they plan to use for the orphanage, she could keep the children at home until they're all grown up and were ready to go out on their own. One of the kids got so sick eating dirt he almost died. They get one bunch of *matooke* every few weeks from a neighbor, and it was late in coming. He was just trying to fill up."

Pauline shook her head, scowling. "Let me know when you go the next time, and I'll give you a hand. Sure hope this thing works out today, because you and I can only help so many people, you know." She brightened. "If we Ugandans would stop breeding like rabbits," she laughed, "AIDS won't hurt anywhere near as bad. When I finally went in to have my tubes tied, the nurse told me Ugandan women have the highest fertility on the continent, and that's going some!" "We could stop if those men would slow down a little," Molly laughed. "When we say no, we get beaten and they go get a woman on the side." "You're telling me," Pauline said, grinning. "My husband was busy even after he got sick. And he used to brag that they never made him use a condom. I tried, but he beat the pulp out of me whenever I brought it up. One time when he was drinking *walagi*[1] he accused me of giving him AIDS. Not worth a darn, men. And a woman's got to make a living. Brewing beer is okay, but you're always expected to deliver the other stuff too."

"So what's this thing about sex with monkeys?" Molly asked, noticing that the men had stopped listening. Pauline smiled. "You know my son Paul is working for the new missionaries in town? Well, he was serving dinner the other night and they were talking about Africans. They don't think Paul knows any English, so they talk right in front of him about everything. They were talking about AIDS and said we got it by making love to monkeys." Molly's eyes were wide. Pauline started laughing. "You know what Paul said about them?" Molly shook her head. "He said he thinks they have sex with turkeys, because after he served them a big turkey dinner at the end of November, he heard so much groaning and moaning that he didn't dare go back to clear the dining room until after they'd gone to bed! Rudeness and ignorance don't respect any color bar, I guess."

"Did you hear about that guy in Masaka who started the tourist business, the one with the sign outside his shop that says 'You Are Now Crossing the Equator. Stop here for Cool Drinks'?" Molly asked. "He set up a sink on either side of the equator, and he shows tourists how the water flushes one way above the line and the other way below. He told me himself that there's no such thing, he just tilted each sink in a different direction. So far they've given him so many shillings that he bought a car." "It's no wonder they think we're crazy—sometimes I think we are too," Pauline said.

"Seen that *National Geographic* in Robina's office?" Molly asked. "That young reporter that came through here to talk to us was so nice, now look what he put in that magazine!" Pauline blushed deeply. "You didn't!" Molly said. "Only once," Pauline said. "In the back of his Land Rover, way out in the country, when I was guiding him to Lyantonde. Don't you ever tell a soul." "What about Carver, that British boy?" Molly asked. "Ask me no question, and I'll tell you no lies," Pauline scowled into her tea. "He had girls all over the district. You know Christine's little boy?" "The baby?" Molly gasped. "No, no, no. The third born, the one that's three. He was nice. He loved the peace and quiet here," Pauline sighed. "People are so afraid to come here, and they're always surprised to find it's so peaceful." "Well, those checkpoints don't make anyone comfortable," Molly said, "especially when they're manned by drunken twelve-year-olds with an AK-47s in their trigger-happy hands."

✻ ✻ ✻

In Africa today, HIV/AIDS has intertwined with crippled economic and social development to rip society apart along every conceivable dimension. While HIV/AIDS has created its own inexorable dynamic, like a massive fire in a very large building that creates its own up- and downdrafts, the building was already shaky, its foundations wracked by the civil strife and poverty familiar to Robina, Pauline, and Molly. Well before the slave trade witnessed by Darwin, Africans had been unmercifully and systematically exploited by outsiders who took what they could with little or no thought to long-term payback. In the mid-1990s, the dreadful synergy of AIDS and nondevelopment intersected and locked in a downward spiral creating what many believe to be a failed continent and tipping the development task from challenging to impossible.[2]

South African Karen Jochelson says that AIDS aggravates an already dim view of Africa's reality and potential, an image of Africa perpetrated since colonial days "as a sick and dying continent, harbouring deadly disease and inhabited by an essentially promiscuous people who are part of a dangerous, wild, natural world and bound by primitive traditions and superstitions." Racist beliefs held by outsiders, like the missionaries in Molly's town, encouraged them to blame the victims, never understanding that life for poor people in Africa is pretty much the same as life for poor people anywhere in the world. Parodying the beliefs of many Americans, the boxer Mohammed Ali asked Ugandan children if they lived in trees when he visited them during his "Rumble in the Jungle" with George Frazier. Otherwise educated and intelligent people believe that AIDS is worse in Africa because Africans have sex with monkeys, jumbling the messages of television programs to connect "Africa," "AIDS," and "monkeys" in a way that reflects their fears of Africans as wild and savage beings.

As we analyze the epidemic in Africa and develop strategies to mitigate its effects, it is critical to understand clearly the forces that set the stage there for the epidemic's horrible impact. When we take a moment to brush aside the mantle of racism inherited from colonial days—shared, tragically enough, even by some Africans themselves—to get a better idea of what Africa is really like and what has happened there over the past 200 years, it becomes very clear why AIDS took off so quickly and why it is worse in Africa than anywhere else in the world.

Columbia University economist and activist Jeffrey Sachs says, "at the root of Africa's poverty lies its extraordinarily disadvantageous geography, which has helped to shape its societies and its interactions with the rest of the world." Africa has the least developed economy of any continent except Antarctica and is the only continent that is almost entirely tropical, with 80 percent of its territory lying between the Tropics of Cancer and Capricorn. Countries that lie outside of this zone in northern and southern Africa are well developed, so much so that they do not seem to be in the same century as the countries that lie between. With the exception of Nigeria, northern and southern Africa are also the only parts of the continent that are densely populated. Only nine countries of Africa's sixty-three have more than 15 million people, despite rapid population growth between 1950 and 1990 during a postindependence recovery from the centuries-long depletion of slavery, labor conscription, and war. Societies with high growth rates have proportionately more children, creating a huge demand for health and education services. Africa's ratio of nonproductive to productive people, children to adults, is the highest in the world, imposing a substantial economic drag. In other regions of the world, population pressure has stimulated invention and new modes of productive activity. Africa has had no "green revolution" in agriculture; when soils are exhausted, farmers move on. Distances between settlements are great, increasing the cost for providing services like healthcare and education, and the domestic market for manufactured goods is small.

Only the very top of Africa's highest mountain ranges get frost, which American expert Naomi Chazan calls "nature's great executioner." Disease parasites, which are never killed in the year round heat, proliferate in both humans and animals, reducing human productivity and agricultural output. People die early deaths, and their capacity for strenuous labor is reduced by parasitic diseases like malaria, sleeping sickness, river blindness, and elephantitis. Diseases are much more difficult to eradicate than in temperate zones, and food production is more difficult because tropical soils are notoriously poor, leached by heavy rains that destroy the particle structure of the topsoil. Plant and livestock development is inhibited because breeds imported from other continents for crossbreeding cannot survive the heat and the pests. Constant heat and humidity, heavy rainfall, and dense vegetation limit road and rail construction and destroy communication systems. Rainfall varies from one year to the next by up to 300 percent and comes in short, torrential bursts, eroding agricultural soil, tearing roads apart, and destroying houses and businesses. There is little flood or deforestation infrastructure, and when it is put in place, it often robs Peter to pay Paul. For example, Ethiopians have long protested the international superpower deals that allow Egypt to drain most of the water from Ethiopia's rivers, lowering the country's agricultural productivity and leaving 60 million people on the brink of perpetual starvation.

Despite relatively low population density, Africans are the most physically varied people in the world. The continent is home to the world's tallest and the world's shortest humans with the entire range of human skin colors and facial shapes. Africans have the most genetic variation because they are the oldest human population and because mortality and adaptive demands are so great. In Africa, disease and environmental pressures have operated to keep the human and parasite gene banks operating at their fullest potential. Two-thirds of Africa's 832 million people still live in rural areas, growing crops and raising livestock, leading lives that are not much different from those of their ancestors hundreds of years ago. Life for most modern Africans is marginal, harsh, and poor, but not as static as it once was. Poverty drives family members to find work off the farm, in manufacturing, mines, and cities. Africa is the least urban of all the continents but has the fastest rate of urbanization, increasing from one-seventh of its total population in 1950 to one-third in 1990 and two-fifths in 2000.

Africa has been the poorest and slowest-growing region of the world since the Industrial Revolution, when its economic situation was better. In 1820 sub-Saharan Africa's production was one-third of Europe's, but by 1992 it was one-twentieth of Europe's. Per capita income was the same as Europe's in 1820, but now fifteen of the world's twenty poorest countries are in the region, where 47 percent of the population lives in abject poverty on less than $1 per day, facing survival margins so tight that any adversity—not to mention a major catastrophe like illness and death from AIDS—can quickly be fatal. Access to services is very uneven, emphasizing a growing separation between the elites and the masses. Several African countries, including Botswana and South Africa, have some of the highest concentrations of wealth in the world. By 1985 agricultural growth rates had declined so precipitously in twenty-two countries that they could no longer feed themselves, and economic growth rates in the 1970s and 1980s were stagnant or negative. Economic declines continued through the 1990s, leaving most countries with staggering foreign debt. Debt, combined with internal economic weakness, forced many countries to hand economic decision making over to the World Bank and International Monetary Fund.

Many countries depend on only one or two farm or mineral products for more than half of their export earnings, creating tremendous economic dependency on a fluctuating world market. These countries have become "enclave economies" dominated by an easily extractable and concentrated source of wealth that has been commandeered by a small elite with little connection to the local population. Exploitation of Africa's natural wealth has always been a harsh business, resulting in colonial and postcolonial atrocities of the worst kind, twisting the political and economic development process of many countries and creating conditions conducive to the wildfire spread of AIDS and other diseases. Gabon's oil, for example, gives it one of the highest gross national products and highest per capita incomes in the region, but its wealth has been siphoned off by elites, leaving most people dirt poor. Following independence, Zaire's Mobutu Sese Seko personally exploited his country's diamond, gold, copper, and cobalt mines, leaving his people in abject poverty and the country with a foreign debt the size of his Swiss bank accounts. Conflict diamonds—diamonds extracted by rebels and renegade governments—fund lawlessness in Sierra Leone, Angola, and the new Democratic Republic of the Congo, and are also thought to fund international terrorist activities. Since the recent discovery of its enormous offshore petroleum reserves, even the tiny Democratic Republic of Sao Tome and Principe, an island off West Africa's coast, is ripe for exploitative development. The two African countries that have successfully controlled AIDS, Senegal and Uganda, lack easily exploitable caches of mineral wealth. Botswana, Namibia, and South Africa since the end of apartheid in 1994 are diamond- and gold-rich countries where the wealth from enclave production has been shared more widely to good effect.

Ghanaian economist George Ayittey says that thanks to constant outside interference, the typical African vehicle of state is hopelessly broken down,

> a motley collection of obsolete, discarded parts scrounged from foreign junkyards [that] operates on borrowed ideology. The carburetor was a gift from Norway and the battery was donated by Austria. The tires came from Britain and China and are mismatched. A headlight is broken and the electric system malfunctions. Turn the ignition switch and the windshield wipers fall off. The engine sputters and belches thick smoke that pollutes the entire country. There are no brakes or shock absorbers (no checks and balances). The fan belt is ripped, which means its cooling system is inoperative. Clutching the wheel of

the state vehicle is a reckless and unskilled egomaniac who proclaims himself "driver for life" and insists that he, and he alone, must be the driver till kingdom come since the vehicle is his own personal property. Aboard are his ministers, cronies, tribesmen, mistresses, sycophants, and other patronage junkies, who, in turn, have brought along their relatives, tribesmen, and friends. A goat has been tied to the rear bumper.

Vehicles like these are not impossible to fix and are driven by poor people all over of the world. "Road monsters," hacked together from the parts of other vehicles, can be found in many developing countries, usually driving at night at great speed without headlights on back roads. Keeping a vehicle like this on the road requires great ingenuity. The rough-and-ready mechanics who jump out of nowhere even in the most far removed parts of the African bush and patch your car with string and water so you can make it back to the capital are a strength and resource all over the continent. As Chazan points out, "perhaps the greatest achievement of African states since independence, especially in light of events in Eastern Europe in the 1990s, has been the fact that they have endured. Even in cases of apparent collapse, most notably Chad and Uganda at the beginning of the 1980s, and Liberia, Rwanda, and Congo in the 1990s, governmental structures have persisted." In postcolonial Africa, many countries realized substantial economic achievements and more than half Africa's population got clean water, electricity, safe sewage, and roads. Education levels increased, and more people had access to radio and television. Despite political unrest, had the AIDS epidemic not occurred, longer-term improvements might have been realized.

✳ ✳ ✳

The evil legacy that brought Africa to its knees was fivefold: slavery, colonialism, labor exploitation in World Wars I and II, governmental distortion, and the Cold War. Unabashed exploitation of the continent was the norm from the early 1600s until independence in the 1960s when African states, ill-prepared for self-rule, were suddenly cut loose by their weakened European masters, who were willing to strike convenient deals with the United States and the Soviet Union to reduce their empires at the end of World War II.

Slavery formally ended with Britain's imposition of antislavery provisions and its crusade to emancipate other colonial populations in the middle of the nineteenth century, prompted by British missionary-explorer David Livingstone's soulful outcry about conditions in Africa. However, the institution of bondage and forced labor did not end until independence in the

1960s, perpetuated by plantation labor, public works, and military conscription during the two world wars. Forced labor did not end legally until 1946 in West Africa, and it continued in Belgian and Portuguese colonies through the next decade.

Slavery has existed in almost every known society. Roughly one-tenth of the English population listed in the Domesday Book of 1086 were slaves, all of continental Europe had slavery, as did indigenous societies in the New World and most parts of Asia, where a quarter to a third of seventeenth- to nineteenth-century populations in Thailand and Burma were enslaved. Slavery still exists in Burma and in several other parts of the world, but nowhere was it as extensive and demographically and socially destructive as in Africa. It is true that Europeans did not introduce slavery to Africa. Indigenous slavery was widespread in precontact Africa and served as the basis for European expansion of the trade. Where population was less dense, chiefdoms prevailed, but where population density was high, more complicated kingdoms held sway over the nobility, extended family groups, and slaves. In northern Nigeria, plantation economies were sustained by bonded labor before the Europeans came on the scene, and slaves had key roles as artisans and domestics, and in the military.

Some historians believe that European slavery actually saved adult males from slaughter by African chiefs and kings, who were interested only in women and children for labor and lineage incorporation. While this may be partially true, many of these slaves faced certain death when they were sold to European traders. Slavery was not only inhumane, but it switched the focus of African leaders from development-oriented trade in legitimate goods to barbarous mutual exploitation. Historian Peter Schwab says that "after about 1650... African production-for-export became a monoculture in human beings." When chiefs partnered with the white slavers, societies were internally divided and traditional life was upended. The slave trade upset the balance of power and undermined the cohesion of many of the ancient centralized states in West Africa. Coastal chiefs raided interior villages to increase their power and, in many cases, to save their own villagers from being taken by the white slavers.

Darwin's picture of slavery's terrors is almost tame compared to the reality of the trade. Chazan says that Europeans "transformed the scale and context of the institution" to get enough labor for New World plantations so that its impact was disastrous. African slaves were needed to replace Native American populations that had been decimated (literally reduced to one-tenth their size) by European conquest. European ships expanded their capacity to meet this demand. Historian Sheldon Watts says that the Portuguese drew on "their privileged access to an apparently inexhaustible source of sturdy servile labor in what is now Angola"[3] and by the 1490s were bringing 1,000 to 2,500 slaves a year to markets in Lisbon, Seville, and the Italian city-states. When sugarcane cultivation was transferred to the New World from the Old, the Portuguese followed the conveniently direct route from Angola to Brazil. Of the 30 million captives "sent down the Path" to coastal collection points in West Africa between the 1670s and the end of the 1800s, half survived, and nineteen of twenty survivors were sent to Brazil. An additional 18 million Africans were traded from east, central and northern Africa through the Islamic and Indian Ocean slave trades between 650 and 1905.

From the mid-1400s to the late 1800s, in addition to the millions of slaves from West Africa who reached foreign ports, another 2 million people lost their lives on the passage between Africa and the Americas. Losses and deaths during the forced march to the coast were probably as high. Conditions were so bad on some New World plantations that 50,000 healthy slaves had to be replaced every twenty years. In Africa, depopulation ranged from gradual, where it did not disrupt the social fabric, to severe, as in Angola, where Chazan says that "intensive slave traffic resulted in depopulation that devastated local communities and undermined subsequent growth." Attempting to escape the trade, substantial numbers of people migrated to the interior, to more remote and inhospitable economic zones, reducing their productivity. Schwab says that the slave trade "robbed Africa of its best and brightest, its farmers and workers, [and] brought about acute economic stagnation." The slave trade took away the same population—young adults who were the most productive members of society—as AIDS, and kept the continent in chaos for four centuries, engulfed in a war of all against all.

The second defining event in the history of sub-Saharan Africa was colonialism. The Scramble for Africa, as the rush for colonial territories in Africa beginning in 1880 has been called, was a "remarkable burst of expansionist energy" that began almost as an afterthought of burgeoning jingoism on the European continent itself. While European powers had gained mightily from their colonial adventures elsewhere in the world, only the Portuguese viewed Africa as a target of colonialism before 1880. Other powers saw Africa as a source of labor to exploit their other, more important possessions until the late 1800s. When the European pressure cooker heated up, colonial territories in Africa became wild cards in a terrible poker game. Peace in Europe was preserved because international rivalries were expressed in the conquest of colonies, so that "if one state acquired a useful block of land somewhere in the wet tropics, this gain would be quickly balanced by counter-annexations by other countries," according to Oliver Ransford, a British colonial doctor who worked in Africa in the 1920s and '30s.

The grab for territories began suddenly. "When I left the Foreign Office in 1880," Lord Salisbury remarked, "nobody thought much about Africa. When I returned in 1885, the nations of Europe were almost quarreling with each other as to the various portions of Africa south of the Sahara they could obtain." In the interim, the balance had been tipped by Belgian King Leopold I, the first European ruler to recognize Africa's commercial possibilities and its vulnerability to exploitation. After failing at colonies in Borneo and the Philippines, he decided that he would not lose his chance of gaining a share of the "magnificent cake of Africa" and enlisted Henry Morton Stanley to cut his piece. Stanley signed the first of a series of treaties with bewildered chiefs starting on June 13, 1880, eventually garnering personal ownership of a million square miles of land for Leopold. Britain had pioneered exploration of the continent and moved fast to protect its interests in the Suez for access to its eastern dominions. It also formalized occupation of coastal West Africa (Ghana) while the French grabbed Dahomey and the right bank of the Congo. Germany claimed Togo, Cameroon, Tanzania, and Namibia.

To avert the dangers of competitive annexation, the United States and every European power except Switzerland met between November 1884 and February 1885 to agree on frontiers of expansion and colonization in Africa. They divided up the land, settled navigation rights, determined levels and procedures of taxation. Ransford says that "compromises were quickly reached and frock coated statesmen joined each other in tracing frontier lines on their maps which carved up the continent in a manner that was without reference to history, geography or ethnic considerations." Europeans thought of Africa as "'vacant,' legally *res nullius*, a no-man's land," up for grabs. According to historian Thomas Parkenham, "in half a generation, the Scramble gave Europe virtually the whole continent, including thirty new colonies and protectorates, 10 million square miles of new territory, and 110 million dazed new subjects, acquired by one method or another." The Scramble was disguised as an effort to humanize Africa and raise it out of the degradation of slavery—caused in large part by the Europeans themselves— but it was really motivated by "dreams of El Dorado" during a slump in European economies that badly needed new resources and markets.

The period of European official colonial domination in Africa was relatively short, only seventy to eighty years, but its impact was devastating. Imperialism meant the introduction of deadly diseases and decimation of native populations forced to extract the wealth of the continent from mines and plantations. Hut taxes, land taxes imposed on the Africans, were so oppressive that local men developed regular migration patterns to avoid them, along with conscription and penalties. Local resistance was common and crushed with armed force. In the Congo, Rwanda, and Burundi, more than 6 million died in Belgian genocide. The Germans issued a *Vernichtungbefehl* (extermination order) against Hereros in South West Africa who revolted against their brutality and drove 20,000 tribesmen out into the desert to die of thirst.

✳ ✳ ✳

When the tensions behind the colonial powers' Scramble for Africa finally ignited in World War I, they turned once again to Africa for soldiers to supplement their fighting forces and African peasants to feed their armies. The end of slavery had created a labor crisis that was met by continuing the institution under other names.[4] The French, Germans, and British had already developed a system to extract native labor for public works and agricultural production and used native troops to control their colonies, but when it became apparent that war in Europe was inevitable, they stepped up recruitment efforts. France had militarized its African colonies more than any other European power and was unique in maintaining universal male conscription from 1912 through 1960 in peace as well as war. While the British, Belgians, and Germans recruited some of their army and police locally and used native troops for defense, France used *Tirailleurs Sénégalais*, Senegalese (African) sharpshooters or riflemen, as an expeditionary force in every corner of its empire. According to historian Myron Echenberg, *"Tirailleurs Sénégalais* paratroopers jumped into the inferno of Dien Bien Phu in 1954." Africans were recruited to become "France's 'black watchdogs of empire' . . . a torturer, bogeyman, and general agent of French coercion," Echenberg says. West Africa Wolof soldiers fought in Madagascar in 1827 and were dispatched across the Atlantic to Martinique and Guyana. France was the only colonial power to bring Africans by the thousands to the trenches of Europe in both world wars.

France brought "men of color" from the French West Indies during the Napoleonic era to serve as officers and soldiers in France's colony of Senegal. The first African troops were formally conscripted in 1820, and by 1823 the first all-African company was formed. Their numbers grew dramatically during France's military occupation from 1890 to 1904 and under civilian rule, until by the beginning of 1914 there were 18,000 men organized in six regiments. Soldiers were purchased as slaves under a system called *rachat*, literally redemption or emancipation through fourteen years of military service. Although *rachat* became an embarrassment—especially when a French trader

named Marbeau, licensed by the governor of Senegal to purchase slaves from
the Portuguese regions of Guinea, was captured en route to Bissao by a
British Anti-Slavery Squadron in the early 1840s—it blurred the lines of
slavery and allowed the French to capture the men they needed. They tried
to attract volunteers, but by 1918, 75 percent of its West African soldiers
were still slave in origin.

After the French suffered severe losses in the first year of World War I,
massive recruitment began that involved almost half of the able-bodied men
in the colony. The number of recruits sent abroad between 1914 and 1918
exceeded all the slaves shipped in French holds from the Senegambia to the
New World during the entire eighteenth century. More than 170,000 West
Africans were conscripted and 140,000 served as combatants on the Western
Front, roughly 5 percent of all males above fifteen years of age. In rural
Senegal between 1914 and 1917, the recruitment methods were "virtually
indistinguishable from slave raids," according to historian Joe Lunn.
Runaways were so numerous that they changed patterns of regional migra-
tion. Repression of revolts caused large-scale population movements in
Guinea; in some parts of Senegal, six people were killed for every one
recruited. Chiefs raided other villages so they could fill their quotas without
disrupting their own villages and turn a profit. If the chiefs failed to comply,
they were imprisoned and the French burned their villages, seized crops and
livestock, took parents of young men hostage, and killed armed resisters.
French administrators also increased hut taxes before the war and requisi-
tioned eight days of *travaux forcé* (forced labor) from all their African
subjects, including the sexual service of African women, who were rotated
every two months or so.

The *Tirailleurs Sénégalais* were brought to France, mixed with French
troops, and fought alongside Canadian and British troops at Vimy Ridge and
the Somme. They were "temporarily amalgamated" with black American
forces—200,000 of whom served in Europe in World War I—in French
trenches in 1918, but after the near collapse of the French army in 1917, they
were dispersed along the front to serve as tactical spearheads for larger French
units. In the last year of the war, they served primarily as assault troops, with
French battalions behind and on their sides to keep them from deserting if
things got hot. According to Lunn, "during the last two years of the war,
many generals sought to spare French lives by sacrificing African ones." More
than one-quarter of the Africans died—31,000 men—a higher proportion
than French troops. Losses among Senegalese combatants were 20 percent
higher than among the French when compared overall (1.3 million of
France's 5 million soldiers and close to three-quarters of their citizens in

uniform died. If infantrymen alone are compared—Africans did not serve in the cavalry, artillery, engineering, or air corps—Senegal lost twice as many men.

When World War I ended, a large portion of the West African army was not demobilized and recruitment continued. By 1920 the standing army of West Africans numbered 55,000, which grew to 110,000 by 1925. France had lost 2 million men in the war, and the West African soldiers filled the "hollow cohorts" of their mother country between 1934 and 1938. The labor loss in their colony's villages caused famine and starvation, but France was so afraid of being overpowered by Germany that it even ignored the protests of its own governor-general in Senegal, who argued that brutal recruitment and labor and food shortages had demoralized the colony and hurt private companies. He warned that the colonies were on the brink of revolt; in fact, there were two armed revolts in Dahomey, one of the French colonies, in 1915–1916. But "France needed soldiers more than peanuts," and the governor-general resigned in protest. He left for the trenches, where he was killed in action in 1918. At that point, Blaise Diagne, a popular Senegalese politician, was named commissioner-general of recruitment and given rank equivalent to the governor-general. He recruited 60,000 Senegalese with almost no armed resistance because the men expected that they would be rewarded with French citizenship. Africans were also being conscripted for two- to three-year stints on public works in the Sudan, but the death rates were so high and the work so hard that military recruitment was preferred.

The African contribution during World War II was even larger than during the first. Africans comprised 9 percent of France's forces in World War II compared to 3 percent in World War I. Seven African divisions totaling 100,000 soldiers joined three other colonial divisions defending the French border in 1939. Up to 48,000 were declared missing when France fell in June 1940, and some 15,000 to 16,000 ended up as prisoners of war in German labor camps in northeastern France. Recruitment under Vichy rule in French West Africa picked up again, and between 1943 and 1945 another 100,000 Africans left for the front. Africans helped the French retake Provence from the Germans in 1944, where they comprised 20 percent of France's total force. Of the more than 200,000 Africans who had gone to Europe, 12 percent ended up dead, *mort pour la France*. Late in the war, when the Allied victory was assured, Africans were removed from their regiments to "whiten" the Free French forces. They were replaced by young French secondary school graduates so they would not be seen in D-Day operations.

Hitler railed against the presence of black Africans in the French army as "pollution" and "negrification" of once-pure French blood, declaring it an insult to have to fight against African forces. Germans continued to denigrate African soldiers after the war, when their component of the occupation army was called the "black shame." Although accusations of atrocities were refuted repeatedly, the African soldiers were eventually removed. The Germans feared the Africans, whom they viewed as an immensely brave, bloodthirsty army of great warriors fiercely loyal to France. Charles Mangin, the French general of the West African forces, liked to tell the story of Sergeant Baba Koulibaly, a six-foot-four inch-tall Bambara who was his personal bodyguard from 1903 to 1922. Early in August 1914 Koulibaly drove off a German patrol of eleven that ambushed the general's motor escort, chased off a second patrol of six Germans, linked up with French cavalry men to ward off another patrol attracted by the noise, and then, unable to gallop off with them because he was a foot soldier, stood alone in the village square. According to Mangin, General de Vaulgrenant found him all alone, leaning on his rifle. "What are you doing here?" asked the general. "I'm occupying the village," he replied.

African troops were described by a contemporary journalist as "headcutters who could, almost singlehandedly, scare *le boche* all the way back to Berlin," and the Germans in turn reviled the French for employing "cannibals," declaring that African resistance around Reims was "conducted by mindless blacks drunk on reserves of brandy and all brandishing the *coupe-coupe*, a big combat knife." Four battalions of *Tirailleurs Sénégalais* were trucked from France to a bend of the Yser River in Belgium to shore up defenses against the German drive to the channel, and after enduring heavy shelling for several days, they were attacked by 40,000 German infantry. Of the 10,000 defenders, only 32 men of the First Senegalese Battalion survived, 100 of the Second, 51 of the Fourth, and half of the Third, but the line had been held. *Tirailleur* Bakary Diallo said a German captive, who saw himself surrounded by *Tirailleurs,* began to shake. "Poor man," said Diallo, "couldn't you have expected this possibility just as well as the gold of glory? May your fear not prevent you from proclaiming in your country, tomorrow, after the battle, the sentiment of justice which will rehabilitate the name of the human race of which we are all savages?" Diallo wrote that "courage in battle has a high value for the *Tirailleurs Sénégalais*. If by some misfortune they were able to see how my insides were churning with fear, I would have lost their esteem forever. . . . Despite my trembling heart, I maintained an exterior of iron."

General Charles de Gaulle was embarrassed by the role the Africans had played in liberating France. He had promised Africans a "new deal" in Brazzaville in 1944, but forgot, Echenberg says, that "without the rank-and-file black African soldier, [French] victories would have been impossible."

Returning African soldiers did not forget, and veterans became a sizable postwar interest group, some with connections to the French socialist movement and the *Ligue des Droits de l'Homme* (Human Rights League). The returnees expected privileges, including pensions and exemption from forced labor. They were allowed to buy guns for hunting. Many maintained modern hygienic practices and retained their taste for meat, cigarettes, and alcohol. Those who had been slaves prior to service were now free men, joining bureaucrats, licensed dealers, diploma holders, and chiefs who could not be penalized arbitrarily for insubordination or disrespect to colonial officials without a hearing. It was an explosive situation. *Ancien combattants* led strikes and work stoppages that reverberated into the interior, but there were no large-scale industries where the labor movement could grow. Returning soldiers led bands of slaves who ran to escape forced labor and organized resistance to the chiefs' demands. In 1950 there were more than a quarter of a million claims for veteran benefits from French West Africa. Violence in Algeria and Madagascar was countered with brutal colonial reprisals as a warning to this group, and West African troops, pared down to a permanent force of 38,000 at the war's end, were used for labor and as strike breakers in France. Although they could be sent to other colonies only if they had volunteered, in 1949, 18,000 *Tirailleurs* were serving in Indochina.

Soldiers returning from both wars also brought with them a variety of diseases that had been unknown in West Africa, drastically increasing local rates of tuberculosis, pneumonia, and sexually transmitted diseases. During campaigns in Africa, the soldiers had been accompanied by their wives, who cooked, collected fire and water, and sometimes even assisted in the fighting. If the soldiers' pay and rations were not enough, they took spoils of conquest from other African households conquered by the French. When not at war, soldiers slipped out of their barracks at night to visit local women for sex and established local households. Prostitutes—"African women dressed in bright silk petticoats and silver bangles, laughing and strumming musical instruments,"—also serviced remote locations in *Bordels Mobiles de Campagne*, according to military historian Anthony Clayton. In military brothels, there were separate services for whites and Africans. Soldiers had to show a pass on entering and were severely punished if they failed to receive prophylactic treatment before leaving. The women underwent daily medical exams. In garrison towns, soldiers were expected to contract semi-permanent liaisons with local women, and in Indochina West African military personnel took a *congai*, or local wife. Despite these efforts, Echenberg says that STDs were rampant and infertility so high that "along with migrant workers, soldiers helped change the course of West African demographic history in the interwar years."

The disruption caused by recruitment and its avoidance, the loss of productive men, the drain of subsistence farmers' yields, and the diseases brought by returnees substantially changed East African history as well. From 1902 to 1964 East Africans were recruited for the King's African Rifles (KAR) from Kenya, Uganda, Tanzania, and Malawi, and soldiers were also recruited to the Somaliland Camel Corps, the Northern Rhodesia Regiment, the Northern and Southern Rhodesian African Rifles, the South African Rifles, and the Royal West African Frontier Force, British West Africa's colonial army. During World War I the KAR included almost 32,000 infantrymen supported by nearly half a million African noncombatant porters. Early recruits were used to expand British territory and subdue other Africans. During World War II 470,000 Africans were in KAR uniform, supported by even larger numbers of laborers. They served extensively in the Asian theater during World War II and were crucial in the defense of the Middle East in the 1940s. Some 100,000 KAR were used in the Burma campaign. In addition, South Africa sent 135,000 white South Africans to fight in East and North African Italian campaigns, along with 70,000 Africans and Coloureds (South Africans of mixed descent) as laborers and drivers. After the war the KAR, led by colonial officers, maintained local order and defended colonial borders, providing "the coercive force that made British rule in East Africa possible," according to historian Timothy Parsons.

As in West Africa, East African soldiers were drawn from the lower classes or, in the most extreme cases, enslaved. Most were unskilled rural men who viewed soldiering as a long-term labor contract, "just like the way people go to the mines in South Africa," as a Malawian veteran put it. Recruitment, as in West Africa, had been actively resisted and substantially disadvantaged the villagers who struggled to maintain livelihoods after the loss of their most productive workers. When heavy demands were also made for agricultural goods to support the European war effort, chaos and suffering resulted, exacerbating the already dismal rural poverty in all British colonies. When the soldiers were not demobilized in the Middle East following Hitler's defeat because the British had no replacement troops, they staged strikes and riots, and disaffection continued when they were not rewarded with good jobs on their return. Pensions were delayed until 1950.

The enslavement and conscription of African soldiers by European powers to extend their imperial designs in the Africa, the Caribbean, and Asia, and their continued conscription to fight in Europe, the Middle East, and Asia during World Wars I and II extended the horror and disruption of slavery through the entire colonial period until just before independence in the 1950s and 1960s. African material resources were also commandeered to meet Europe's needs during both wars, an expropriation so severe it endangered the lives of many Africans, who could not hold back enough food to feed themselves. Entire agricultural systems were subverted to European war efforts, and village social systems were turned upside down, creating famine conditions in Kenya, Tanzania, Nigeria, and French West Africa. Resources that might have been used for long-term, sustained development were drained away from the entire continent for European use. Africa's participation in the European war effort through the first half of the twentieth century left them unprepared for independence and wide open to the spread and impact of diseases, including, most significantly, curable STDs and HIV/AIDS.

❊ ❊ ❊

According to African expert Bill Freud, World War II "dramatically exposed the poverty of Africans to Europe. Dependent colonies with limited infrastructures and populations producing little beyond their barest needs could offer little assistance to the mother countries."[5] What better solution than to set them free? In the late 1950s colonies in North Africa and Ghana were the first to gain their independence. By 1960 France's extensive colonial empire had been dismantled, and Nigeria attained its sovereignty from Britain. Five years later, more than thirty states were independent. Spain gave up its interests in Equatorial Africa in 1968, and finally let go in North Africa after the death of General Francisco Franco in 1975. Portugal held onto its colonies until a revolution at home in 1974 triggered colonial liberation wars. British rule ended in Rhodesia in 1980, bringing their presence on the continent to an end. Namibia gained independence from South Africa in 1990, and in 1994 South Africa completed its transition to multiracial democracy.

When colonialism came to an end, the African political map reflected European ambitions rather than the geographical and social realities of the African continent. Colonial boundaries had not coincided with precolonial states, tribes, or alliances; arbitrary divisions by colonial authorities left some states with no natural resources and others with a great many. When colonial rulers established control, they overlaid Africa's complex social institutions and governing structures with a foreign institutional framework that governed by playing one party against the other. Colonial rule also had weakened economic structures by giving precedence to cash crops over subsistence production, leaving many areas vulnerable to persistent famine and starvation.

African economies were geared to production for external consumption, creating a legacy of external dependence. When those economies were brought into the world system by colonial powers at independence, they were deliberately subordinated to European needs, leading to lopsided economic systems that were highly vulnerable to external shocks, economies dependent on one export crop whose value fluctuated on the world market. Many free African states still are economically manipulated to serve the interests of other states in the global arena.

Postindependence governments found themselves running very distorted states. While mechanisms for extraction of mineral, agricultural, forest, and other resources were highly developed, systems for redistributing resources, such as healthcare and education, were almost nonexistent. Military and police forces were strong, but ordinary civil participation had been discouraged, so that "efforts to democratize Africa stood in stark contrast to the authoritarian patterns of government laid down during colonial rule," according to African expert Naomi Chazan. "The power apparatus inherited at independence was aloof and surprisingly weak, primarily concerned with issues of domination rather than legitimacy." There were few educated Africans with political experience, and most people were illiterate. In Ghana, which had the best educational institutions at independence, 70 percent of the citizenry was illiterate. Colonial powers had created a very thin stratum of educated servants, new elites who became "the direct inheritors of the colonial mantle," says Chazan.

Local competition for power was strong, and African leaders who had little experience in creative political problem solving wanted to consolidate and centralize their power, reduce competition, and strengthen the ruling party. Now in charge of their economies, they could reward cooperation with state resources. Almost immediately, new governments in Kenya, Uganda, Malawi, Zambia, Ghana, Côte d'Ivoire, and Sierra Leone rewrote their constitutions to eliminate legal "roadblocks" to strong centralized rule. In Guinea, Uganda, Angola, and Mozambique, opposition parties were forcibly suppressed, and by the early 1960s most opposition leaders were in jail or exiled. Côte d'Ivoire's president Felix Houphouet-Boigny said that single-party rule sanctioned the unity that already existed in the country, while Ghana's Kwame Nkrumah argued that multiparty democracy led to divisiveness and reduced national economic integration. To Tanzania's Julius Nyerere, the one-party system reflected Africa's traditions and norms of consensus, an argument still used by Yowero Museveni, Uganda's president, to resist multiparty democracy, although open, fair single-party elections have been held there regularly since 1989.

New university graduates were co-opted into the civil service and often rewarded with salaries that were forty to one hundred times greater than the norm. By 1970, 70 percent of all formal wage earners on the continent were government employees whose salaries consumed at least 50 percent of government budgets. In Tanzania, the economy grew by 3.9 percent between 1966 and 1976 while the civil service expanded by 13.3 percent per year. Civil service employees "ate their offices," developing unofficial ways to line their pockets. In many sectors, state-owned quasi-governmental businesses, or "parastatals," proliferated, and even where there was private competition, dominated through favorable regulation. These parastatals created employment and rewards for civil servants, so their growth was phenomenal in the 1960s and 1970s; most have now been privatized or closed because they were unprofitable and inefficient.

Without checks and balances, African leaders survived by balancing the party, army, and civil service against one another. With the exception of Gambia and Botswana, Chazan says the "coercive apparatus grew alongside the bureaucratic," and soldiers became a political force in their own right. Military expenditures increased from 1.8 percent of gross national product in 1963 to 2.9 percent in 1980 and are still growing; Africa's share of world arms imports increased from 4.6 percent in 1971 to 18.8 percent in 1980. In some states, Chazan says, the army is well-disciplined and "not prone to preying on innocent citizens to supplement their incomes," but in others "faulty lines of command, inadequate salaries, and raw ambition have allowed soldiers...to become, themselves, the cause of indiscriminate lawlessness." The army undermined the state that had created it in Liberia, Somalia, Ethiopia, Rwanda, and the Congo. With power consolidated around the government or the army, other social groups and communities and even party diehards often were kept outside official power circles. In the rush to consolidate postcolonial rule, the state "pushed society out," Chazan says, creating "Big Africa" and "Little Africa," where the only means of access to state power was co-optation or violence. African states had come to resemble the colonial powers they had thrown off.

With the start of the Cold War, the United States and the Soviet Union moved in quickly to replace retiring British, French, Italian, German, and Portuguese landlords, extending "ethnic and tribal divisions so that their own interests could be served," according to African analyst Peter Schwab. The competition was fierce, and tribes or nationalities not co-opted by

U.S.-financed or Soviet-supported leadership were left out in the political cold. The U.S. Central Intelligence Agency helped get rid of Patrice Lamumba, Zaire's first prime minister, legitimizing Mobutu Sese Seko as president and propping him up until the 1990s. "Colonization was replaced by a form of Cold War neocolonialism," Schwab says, and elites who could not be controlled were dismissed. The superpowers' local clients received another benefit: billions of dollars' worth of support for their armies and advanced munitions, including heavy weaponry. Since favored tribes had been socialized by their European partners to view rival ethnic groups as alien, when constraints on political violence dissolved with the departure of the Europeans, "the violence that often accompanied the ensuing struggles for indigenous control or superpower hegemony was awesome and destructive."

With the fall of the Soviet bloc and the end of the Cold War in the early 1990s, African players were unceremoniously abandoned by their former partners, who felt no sense of responsibility for their past dealings with the continent. African leadership had been corrupted, armies had been built, antagonisms had been encouraged, and many African states had been turned into battlegrounds. A middle class had never developed, because there were no institutional structures in place outside the government or military where citizens could develop wealth and power. African states that served as strategic pawns in the Cold War paid a severe price in exploitation and loss of opportunities for democratization.

Many African leaders have found that their European and American partners continue to help them create other devastating problems. Not only have they received poor guidance from bilateral aid agencies and their World Bank and International Monetary Fund economic experts, but many foreign advisors have been primarily interested in extracting as much as they can from Africa's rich natural environment. Corporate interests have raped countries in the process of extracting oil, timber, and other wealth. In Nigeria, exploitation of Nigerian oil by Chevron and Royal Dutch/Shell has left their delta region a smoldering ruin. In response to local resistance, the companies pulled out, leaving exploding gas pipelines that have killed hundreds of people and irreversible environmental pollution. In other countries, outsiders who stand to benefit from chaotic conditions have deliberately provoked or prolonged conflicts, so they could grab diamonds, emeralds, gold, and other resources. Even neighboring states have played a role. Preapartheid South Africa perpetuated conflicts in Angola and Mozambique so the foothold of the African National Congress in neighboring states would remain weak.

African countries surrounding the Democratic Republic of the Congo have contributed heavily to perpetuating the conflict there.

Despite these difficulties, the African development picture is less dismal than that painted by many recent critics. Many African countries show signs of emerging from the chaotic postcolonial period and building viable states. But African leaders must overcome a number of other trenchant structural problems to development, including tribalism, uneven regional development, and structural bias against women. To outsiders, tribalism is undoubtedly the most horrifying, entrenched, and difficult characteristic of African traditional society to overcome if modern states are to be built. Ethnic groups in Africa often are portrayed as primordial, but ethnic awareness or tribal identity is a relatively recent phenomenon. Colonial governments consolidated autonomous ethnic groups that lived near one another in order to simplify their administration. In some cases, they even created ethnic groups for administrative purposes. For example, Belgian colonial authorities grouped together the Luhya in Zambia and the Ngala, who lived along the Zaire River, for purposes of taxation. Worse, colonial administrations often pitted relatively peaceful groups against one another, creating long-lasting ethnic rivalries for power. Hutu living in the north and southern sections of Burundi did not perceive of themselves as a group until the Belgians encouraged Tutsis to unite against them in 1972 as a common enemy.

Ethnic self-definition emerged in a relatively short time through colonial interventions and the intense competition over power, status, and economic resources during the late colonial and postcolonial periods. Because of their recent origins, many ethnic groups are not homogeneous or cohesive, and they have diverse interests, values, and commitments. For an ethnic group to behave like an organized interest group, leaders must negotiate common positions and build internal coalitions. Many presumably rock-hard ethnic groups, such as the Kikuyu and Luo in Kenya, the Yoruba of Nigeria, and the Shona in Zimbabwe, are riddled internally by interclan, age-set, gender, and geographic competition.

Except in their most extreme expressions, ethnic groups in Africa function the same way as ethnic groups did in the United States in the late 1800s and early 1900s, when ethnicity served as a rallying cry to organizing the poor and gain political access. In Africa, ethnic identity is still "a useful instrument for mobilizing and aggregating interests in competition with other ethnic, occupational and business groups for state-controlled political and economic

resources," Chazan says. Even Africa's most notorious strongmen—Jomo
Kenyatta in Kenya, Ghana's Kwame Nkruma, and Houphouet-Boigny of
Côte d'Ivoire—responded to pressures for equitable allocation among subre-
gions and for the inclusion of "outsider" representatives in cabinets and ministry positions when ethnic groups organized to press their case. Where
internal government checks and balances were missing in early governments,
ethnic rivalries could check centralization.

Within countries, severe imbalances also exist between cities and rural
areas, and among regions. By exploiting areas of the country with the most
resources and neglecting others, colonial regimes laid the basis for regional
differences, stratifying opportunities within countries that African policymakers cannot easily alter. Disparities often are reinforced by aid agencies
whose resources are directed into certain regions by government bureaucrats
or politicians interested in benefiting their home areas by manipulating the
"pork barrel" that also powers regional politics in the United States. In the
end, it is "small farmers who largely underwrite the expansion of industry,
parastatals, state farms, bureaucracy, military, and urban life-styles," says
Chazan, but their demise now imperils everyone.

Gender inequities are linked to this bias against small farmers.[6] The poorest peasants are predominantly female. Women comprise 70 percent of
Africa's subsistence agricultural workforce and are a class in themselves. Their
lack of gender consciousness hinders efforts to organize them to influence
national politics, where they are generally underrepresented. Women also
suffer economic discrimination, although they are central to the economy,
responsible for 50 percent of animal husbandry, 78 percent of food production, 80 percent of food processing, 80 percent of fuel preparation and water
gathering, and 90 percent of brewing in Africa as a whole. Women are the
beasts of burden, the water pipes, the plows and threshers, but in many countries have no right to own property and have little say over the course of their
lives and futures, no legal existence outside of what they draw from being one
man's daughter or another man's wife. In most of sub-Saharan Africa, 40 to
50 percent of the formal labor force is female, but the proportion of women
who work is close to 100 percent. Unlike men, they will bury their pride and
do whatever job is available to feed their families. Women employed outside
the home work 20 percent longer than men, and 30 to 40 percent more
when household chores are added. Most women are locked into work in
subsistence agriculture, petty trading, low-paying and menial work like
collecting garbage, cleaning toilets, and factory work because they lack education, although the proportion of women who are literate has increased
from one-third in 1980 to nearly half in 1999.

Gender inequities, established through long-standing practice to suit the social orders of traditional agrarian societies, become dysfunctional as societies modernize and change. Severe gender disparities in Africa leave women poor and dependent on men for cash, creating incentives for exchange of sex for money. "I'm not a prostitute," one Ugandan woman told me. "He is an old friend and brings me salt. He brings me sugar, too, and when I need shillings for the children's school fees, I can count on him." Many indicators of women's status are going down, not up, and "many women find themselves more burdened, more impoverished, and more on their own economically than in the past," Chazan says, leaving them even more vulnerable to HIV infection. While the interaction of women's low status and the spread of HIV/AIDS has been widely recognized for more than ten years, only Uganda, South Africa, Mozambique, Namibia, and Botswana have taken decisive action to change destructive inequality because men control the political machinery. After a visit to several African countries in January 2003, the UN Special Envoy for AIDS Stephen Lewis said "women are at the center of the pandemic, as they are acutely vulnerable to infection on the one hand, doing all the care-giving for the sick and the orphans on the other. [But I] saw precious little evidence of efforts at women's empowerment, sexual autonomy or gender equality. And there was certainly no effort whatsoever to relieve their unfair share of the burden. In fact, male hegemony was ubiquitous."

Over recent years, George Ayittey says, two Africas have developed: "Big Africa," leadership elites hitched to the international development framework, and "Little Africa," the Africa of the countryside and small urban neighborhoods. Whether Big Africa works or not, Little Africa remains a solid society that continues to function beneath the chaos, plodding on no matter what the difficulties. This is the Africa of Pauline, Molly, and Robina, the Africa that survives insult after insult, the Africa that has coped with innumerable epidemics in the past and will continue to cope with AIDS in the future. Despite setbacks and inequities, Little Africa is probably considerably better off today than it was during or prior to colonialism.

The "myth of Merrie Africa," popular during the colonial period, claimed that "the rules and regulations of every African Community leave no ground for idle women, prostitutes, or vagabonds, and create no possibility for the existence of waifs and strays, no Barnado's Homes, no Refuge for the Destitute grace the cities because the conditions producing them are absent," says English historian John Iliffe. Although "Merrie Africa" was Victorian propaganda, it had real roots in African social organization. "There were no poor and rich," a South African wrote, "the haves helped those who were in want.

No man starved because he had no food; no child cried for milk because its parents did not have milk cows; no orphan or old person starved because there was nobody to look after them. No, these things were unknown in ancient Bantu society." In rural areas extended family groups are still the main production unit, three to five generations of kin working the fields, maintaining their compounds, and caring for their members throughout their lifetime. "In this type of community," a UN Regional Advisor on Social Welfare wrote in 1972, "no one can be labeled as poor because the group usually shares what they have. There is no competition, no insecurity, no big ambitions, no unemployment [severe underemployment instead] and thus people are mentally healthy. Deviation or abnormal behavior is almost absent."

Communities in Little Africa absorb the impact of poverty because "in rural areas, the extended family and the clan assume the responsibility for all services for their members, whether social or economic. People live in closely organized groups and willingly accept communal obligations for mutual support. The sick, the aged and children are all cared for by the extended family," Iliffe says. As Molly's story shows us, these structures still exist today, but their capacity is severely limited by the poverty of the people that support them. A study sponsored by the UN Children's Fund (UNICEF) in Uganda in the early 1990s showed that the nutritional status of orphans and nonorphans was the same within families, but that families with large numbers of orphans had decidedly lower overall nutritional status than those without. Studies in Zambia and South Africa through the 1990s showed that families were willing to take in orphans if they could afford it but that the whole fostering family suffered days without food if they were poor. Traditions of family and community self-help that the UN Advisor found in 1972 still prevail despite severe constraints arising from the HIV/AIDS epidemic, but as more people become sick and die, the weak will outnumber the strong and the entire system may collapse.

�֍ �֍ ✖

Conservative neoliberal critics say that bad leadership, corruption, and selfish elitism devoid of statesmanship have led Africa to the brink of an irreversible decline. Liberal observers claim that the continent has been ripped nine ways to Sunday by greedy colonial imperialists who stripped away everything the land had to offer with no regard for the terrible long-range consequences and no intention to pay it back, and who continue even today to extract everything they can working through native elites. What slavery, labor conscription, and the Cold War started, the World Bank, AIDS, and poverty will finish. But asking if Africa's problems are internal or external is more than academic. Problems come from both sources, reflecting the growing pains of societies yanked out of relatively undeveloped social conditions into the harsh light of the modern world, destined to move from the medieval world into the modern era in less than half a century.

Relationships with the outside world have cost Africa dearly in death and forced labor, lost productivity and resources, continual chaos, dysfunctional political and economic systems. "For more than five centuries, first Europe, then the United States and the Soviet Union have done what they could to eviscerate Africa and its people," says Schwab. Some have called for reparations, like those given by the United States to Native Americans, but "they will hardly compensate for the paralysis imposed history has caused in Africa," he claims. Others have called for a truce. Who cares, they say, where this started? If it is allowed to continue, it amounts to deliberate genocide. Let's at least forgive Africa's staggering debt so it can keep the money it now sends to the developed world and use it to protect its poor. A third group says that the worst faults of African leadership created during colonial years are still being perpetuated by Africa's interaction with the global economic system. The "bad driving" of postcolonial African leaders is still being encouraged by their outside partners, both of whom are busy realizing only their own private interests. They are lining their pockets by heavily mortgaging the future of the continent, creating a debt the rest of us will struggle to repay in the future. Whatever one believes is the cause of Africa's failure to develop, it is clear that AIDS is the reward. But it is not the only reward Africa has received, as we will see in the next chapter, which looks at the history and distribution of other diseases on the continent and their relationship to colonialism and AIDS.

CHAPTER FOUR

Epidemic Rules, Part 1: Causes and Conditions

Cholera reached continental Europe from the Far East for the first time in 1830, the year before Darwin left on the *Beagle*, and severe epidemics were raging in several English cities just as the ship departed. Busy preparing for his trip, Darwin paid little attention to the uproar this "new" disease was causing. He was very disappointed to learn that word about the frightening epidemic had traveled faster than the ship and that his long-anticipated visit to Tenerife, the ship's first planned port of call in the Canary Islands after departing Plymouth, had been canceled because the consul in Santa Cruz would not let the ship dock. Before signing up for the voyage, Darwin had hoped to stage his own collecting foray to the Canaries. "I talk, I think, & dream of a scheme I have almost hatched of going to the Canary Islands," he told a university friend, "I go and gaze at Palm trees in the hot-house and . . . I will never be easy till I see the peak of Tenerife and the great Dragon tree," he wrote his sister Caroline. Hearing that it would take twelve days for the *Beagle*'s quarantine to clear, Captain Fitz Roy headed for Cape Verde instead. "Oh misery, misery . . . we have left perhaps one of the most interesting places in the world," Darwin complained.

Although epidemics were very common in Europe, Darwin had lived primarily in rural areas on his family's private estates, protected from the many communicable disease epidemics that ravaged London and other European cities. Medical responses to cholera and other epidemics were very limited. The connection between cholera and bad water was not identified until 1849, and the cholera bacterium was not discovered until 1883. Darwin had been protected from the personal tragedy of disease until shortly after he married his cousin, Emma Wedgwood. In January 1839 he began to suffer the sustained debilitation of Chagas disease, contracted when he was bitten in Chile by a large black insect, the *Benchuca*. Chagas, caused by a parasite similar to one that causes sleeping sickness in Africa, afflicts more than 18 million South Americans today. Fighting crushing headaches, fever, stomach cramps, insomnia, and depthless fatigue that could not be properly diagnosed, Darwin worked five hours a day in his secluded country house in Kent to back up his theory of evolution with so much evidence that no one could refute it.

When all three of his daughters, Anne, Henrietta, and Elizabeth, caught scarlet fever in 1849, disease began to have an even greater impact on his life. His eldest daughter, Anne, never fully recovered, and in October 1850 the family went on a therapeutic holiday to the seaside resort of Ramsgate. Anne was nine at the time, and her father's favorite child. Darwin had monitored her growth in his journals ever since her birth, noting "how neatly Annie takes hold in proper way of pens and pencils" when she was only fourteen months old. When the sea cure and visits to doctors did not work, he resolved to take her for the cure at Malvern, whose waters had relieved his illness. Anne soon developed a fever and did not respond to the doctor's physics of camphor and ammonia, which made her vomit bright green fluid. She rallied, making Darwin "foolish with delight," but died two days later. Darwin and Emma wept together bitterly, and he was repeatedly overwhelmed with grief. "We have lost the joy of the household, and the solace of our old age. Oh that she could now know how deeply, how tenderly we do still & shall ever love her dear joyous face."

In the months following her death, Darwin's skepticism about the existence of God, awakened by his speculations on natural selection, grew even stronger. He threw himself into his work to deaden his grief and completed one of the last volumes of his extended study of barnacles. His newest child, Horace, was born only three weeks after Anne's death, and a few months later, the whole family went to see Joseph Paxton's Crystal Palace, a great glass cathedral filled with the wonders and accomplishments of Victorian England. Then Darwin met the young and ambitious Thomas Henry Huxley, who erupted onto the London scene after spending four years pent up as a surgeon-naturalist on the HMS *Rattlesnake*. In no time at all Huxley had become known for his anatomical essays, was named to the Royal Society, and received the Royal Medal. The two men became fast friends, and Huxley also befriended the rest of Darwin's circle of confidants.

Painstakingly, slowly, Darwin was accumulating the growing body of evidence he needed for his theory of evolution in special journals, where he also recorded the results of interviews and surveys of plant and animal breeders who systematically bred the changes created by accident in nature. He had roughed out a 240-page "abstract" of the idea in 1844, but set it aside after widespread attacks that same year on Robert Chambers for suggesting the idea of species change in his loosely-documented *Vestiges of the Natural History of Creation*. Darwin saw how dangerous it was to launch a boat against the current until he had his sails in trim, commenting to a friend that admitting to a belief in species change was "like confessing to a murder." His voyage had produced what was for him incontrovertible geological and biological proof that the earth had traveled through millions of years of change and that the human species itself was a product of this change. But he knew the scientific community would require much more evidence to accept the idea of evolution.

Darwin continued to delay until lightning struck so close to home that he was finally forced to take action. On a June 1858 morning, he received a package from Ternate, an island halfway between Celebes and New Guinea. It was from Alfred Russel Wallace and contained a handwritten essay that "line by line, spelled out virtually the same theory of natural selection that Darwin believed was his alone." Darwin had been trumped. He wrote Lyell that natural selection, the work of his lifetime, was for naught, and forwarded Wallace's essay as proof. In his darkest hour, another crisis struck. Daughter Henrietta, then fifteen, came down with a sore throat. The Darwins feared diphtheria, a new disease that had invaded Britain from France. Their son George's headmaster wrote to say the boy had measles, and the next day, their two-year-old, Charles, came down with a fever. Lyell and Hooker proposed that Darwin's and Wallace's papers both be read at the July 1, 1858 meeting of the London Linnean Society so the members could decide who had come up with the idea first, but as Darwin sat up the night before with the sick baby on his lap, he could not decide what to do.

Before Darwin could reply to the proposal, baby Charles became violently ill, getting progressively worse by the hour. Scarlet fever had taken three children in Darwin's village and was sweeping young lives away all over Britain. While three of Darwin's other children had survived it, baby Charles was suffering so badly that Emma and Charles were happy to see him go to his rest on June 28. "It was with the most blessed relief to see his poor innocent face resume its sweet expression in the sleep of death," Darwin later wrote a friend. That night he hastily assembled a bundle of his writings and sent them to Hooker just in time for the Linnean Society meeting. Included was his earlier draft of the *Origin of the Species*, written in 1844, and related correspondence that demonstrated his precedence over Wallace.

❋ ❋ ❋

"Speaking of sinks, here comes a drain that always goes the wrong way," muttered Pauline. Molly glanced in the direction of her nod. "Ugh. It's Wallace Nyumba." "I think we can sneak out the back door before he sees us." They paid Josephine, who shook her head and rolled her eyes toward the blue branches. "Leaving me alone with that guy?"

Molly and Pauline slipped out the back past the latrines and picked their way toward the road through Josephine's chicken pen. "That man," Pauline said, "has to be one of the biggest bores in God's creation. Have you heard his latest lecture on AIDS yet?" "The one he gives all the journalists about how it started on 'Witchcraft Island'?" "Oh, no, not the old theory," Pauline laughed. "He's got a new one. The Tanzanian trader that sold Juliana—you remember that beautiful *kanga* cloth?—he had sex with women who couldn't pay and gave it to them all, starting with one in Lukunyu." "I thought it came from Regina, the prostitute on Busungwe Island. The Kyebe chief said that she infected all the men from Lukunyu and Kasensero."

"Well, I know how I got mine," Pauline said grimly. "Just one man, my dear departed husband. I think he had sex with every prostitute from Kagera to Lyantonde. You know those big men from the north can't keep it in their pocket. Obote, Okello, Amin, Our dear presidents. None of them came close to controlling themselves."

"I always thought Amin had syphilis," Molly said. "But it could have been anyone right after the war. Things were so upside down, everyone trying to make a buck. We had a little bit of everything then. Cholera, malaria, and so many venereal diseases you couldn't tell one from another. I heard a story about some prostitutes north of Bukoba who had a terrible VD in 1981 and were so weak they couldn't walk to the hospital. You know those Haya girls down there made all their money in Nairobi and came back to Tanzania to buy farms. Wherever it started, Tanzania, Uganda, wherever, it sure didn't waste anytime. I think I must have fallen asleep between 1984 and 1986, because there was nothing here when I went to bed and everybody had it when I woke up."

"Not you, though," said Pauline. "You were one of the lucky ones. You got out of here during the war." Molly had spent most of the war years in Kenya, so Pauline told her how the Tanzanian People's Defense Force had responded after Amin's soldiers killed 1,500 Tanzanians just across the border in Kagera in May 1978. "Things weren't going so well here after he threw the Indians out, so he thought he'd start a little war to distract us," she commented. "The Ugandan soldiers raped the women and looted the local towns, capturing 1,000 prisoners of war to work at a labor camp in Kalisizo. They even butchered most of the elephants in Queen Elizabeth Park to feed the troops.

"But it wasn't long before Amin knew he had stepped over the wrong line," Pauline continued. "Nyerere had been watching him and hated everything about him. He called him an oppressor and a 'black fascist,' but Amin got revenge by publicly executing some Tanzanian students who were studying at Makerere. Even though there was a cholera epidemic in Dar es Salaam that year, Nyerere mobilized 45,000 soldiers by November. They took the Kyaka bridge, crossed over, and set up camp in three villages. Sleepy little places that went from a few hundred to thousands of people overnight. They took the Mutukula border post in January, then marched to Minziro, where Amin had massacred almost everybody. By that time, Amin had his artillery positioned in Simba Hills—you know that place just south of Masaka—and Katera near the lake was occupied by Amin's troops and vehicles. The Tanzanians headed straight across the swamp—fifteen miles in three days—and took the hill, then had no trouble chasing Amin back through Kyotera to Masaka and on to Kampala. Boof! Our noble leader was out by June 3, and the celebrations—they'd been going on for five months already—swung into full gear. Do you know that guy really had no feelings at all? He killed his little son and ate his heart so he could increase his own strength."

"Some kind of animal, he was," Molly said. "Someone told me that in the year after the war, there were a lot of children were born with Tanzanian names." "A lot of kids didn't know who their father was back then," Pauline replied. "We had a whole generation who didn't know right from wrong. Things went so crazy, there was rape and murder and torture everywhere. The British condemned Amin because he condoned wholesale rape of all our women. Thousands of people ended up floating in the Nile because of his 'accidents.' It's no wonder my husband thought anything he wanted to do was all right. He was in the liberation force, and he stayed in Kampala for weeks. I had to celebrate by myself," she laughed.

"Look—there's Robina!" Molly pointed at the troop carrier coming up the road from Mutukula. They've had lots more robberies and kidnappings near Kasensero these days." "Down there? I thought everybody was dead by now," Pauline laughed. "Oh, no. I was down there the other day with Robina to see about their orphan report and it's still going strong. There are a lot of young men coming in from Masaka to take over the black market trade. Coffee, tires, batteries, blankets, you name it."

"And a lot of women in slinky little dresses working the bar girl scene," Pauline said. "I met one girl whose mouth was so full of thrush—it's like a creamy paste—that she could hardly breathe. Her face was covered with sores, and she had lost so much weight she looked like a skeleton. She begged me to take her babies out of there, and one of them looked like it had Slim too. The village committee promised to let me know if she dies, but so far I haven't heard a thing. Maybe Robina will know something." The district administrator had jumped down from the troop truck's high front seat and as her officer saluted, she turned and walked toward her house. Molly and Pauline picked up their pace to see her before the crowd of supplicants waiting on her front porch realized she had come home.

✳ ✳ ✳

Epidemics are one of the strongest forces in nature, acting throughout history to shape human choices and lives in every corner of the world. While wars may take precedence in our thinking, microbes are definitely our fiercest competitors. They have literally changed the world, and have done it many times over in very dramatic ways. They have ravaged continents, making way for conquering armies, and then turned around to devastate the would-be conquerors, showing little concern for either party. They have lost empires and gained them, killed kings, poets, artists, and statesmen, humbled churches and changed the direction of religion—Christianity, Islam, Hinduism, and Buddhism—with no regard to the content of theology, leveled entire economic systems, and made way for new forms of social organization. Epidemics have made fortunes and lost them, destroyed the rich and elevated the poor, created new art styles and fashions, and given us the plots of some of our most stirring romantic literature. AIDS is already making its own changes, so there is clearly much to be learned from the thousands of pages of scholarship on past epidemics. Here we will take a look at some of the broader "rules" that govern the behavior of epidemics, and in chapter 5, we will look at responses. AIDS researchers have focused on only two great epidemics in history for comparison, the Black Death of 1347 and the influenza epidemic of 1918, but our vision about epidemics becomes much less blurry if we look at the whole sweep of epidemics through human history. By taking this perspective, the broader evolutionary purpose of epidemics becomes clear.

In the 1870s Louis Pasteur, the father of microbiology and immunology, boasted that it was within "the power of man to make parasitic maladies disappear from the face of the globe."[1] In 1967 the U.S. surgeon general,

William Stewart, declared that we had "closed the book on infectious disease." The 1960s was a decade prone to large statements, but, in retrospect, U.S. president John Kennedy's challenge to put a man on the moon turned out to be a much more reasonable proposition. Even today, thirty-five years after we supposedly "closed the book" on infectious diseases, epidemics of tuberculosis, cholera, malaria, yellow fever, Ebola, Marburg, and SARS rage through developing countries year after year. HIV is only the most powerful among a number of predatory microbes, peers that have threatened us continuously since we separated from apes on the evolutionary tree.

Epidemics are extremely common events and were common all over the globe until the 1950s, when industrialized countries began successfully applying the newly developed technology of antibiotics to treat infectious diseases, reduce postoperative infections, and even treat animals in our food chain. Until AIDS came along in the 1980s, epidemics remained common only in developing countries that have not yet completed the "demographic transition," countries where death rates and birth rates are still high, a transition developed countries completed early in the twentieth century. Since developing countries are home to more than 80 percent of the world's population, the triumph of humans over disease declared by the surgeon general in 1967 was a very limited one indeed. But diseases are not "natural" in certain places because humans are inherently different. Their distribution is determined by technology and wealth. Developing countries are in the situation developed countries faced a century or more ago, where high fertility is necessary to offset dreadfully high mortality. Barely two children in three manage to survive the first year of life, and hardly more than half survive to the age of five. Epidemics caused the same kind of mortality in developed countries until 1950.

While AIDS may be the first "disease of globalization," it is not the first global disease. Humans have not been very successful in controlling the spread of diseases among countries and continents; to the contrary, they have been a major force in their spread. Globalization is just the latest version of the long-distance journeys taken by disease ever since humans took their present form. Our most persistent pathogens originated when the first humans made their great migrations out of Africa to the Middle East, Europe, Asia, and the New World tens of thousands of years ago. Since that time epidemics have raced across connected landmasses with frightening speed even before the invention of the sailing ship, railroad, or automobile. When epidemics came to the end of one continent, human beings more often than not obliged them by carrying them to the next, a fact that was as true of the earliest recorded epidemics in history as it is of the latest scourges. Like its predecessors, the Great Plague of Athens in 431 B.C. and the Roman Plague of

164 A.D., the third great European Plague was carried by rats that gained free passage on ships to Constantinople in 542 A.D. from Egypt and Syria. It made its way across Europe to Spain with Muslim conquerors, raced to France, Germany, and Italy, and migrated to England in 664. By the time it was done, it had cut Europe's population in half. The Black Death of 1347 to 1350 came from Asia via the Silk Road through the Middle East to North Africa, made its way to Italy by ship, then worked its way up the continent, killing one-third of all the humans in its path.

The skin disease, yaws, was carried to Europe with Columbus's sailors in 1492. After it mutated into syphilis, it was spread through Europe with frightening speed by mercenary soldiers, rearing its ugly head in Hong Kong only ten years later. Typhus, another rodent-borne disease like the plague, was introduced to Europe from Asia when the Venetians attacked the Turks in Cyprus, and became epidemic by 1489. The unwashed, undisciplined, malnourished armies of sixteenth- and seventeenth-century Europe were the perfect vector for transmitting typhus all over Europe (along with syphilis), building up the infection pool so much that it persisted continuously in Europe until World War I. Typhus also traveled to the Middle East and Asia, where it caused major epidemics in less than twenty years. Smallpox has terrorized the world many times over since it first appeared in settled agricultural communities in 8,000 B.C. Tuberculosis migrated from cattle to humans in the earliest years of settled agriculture in the Fertile Crescent, carried from there to other continents during the earliest human migrations.

The global circulation of diseases was greatly facilitated by the breathtaking extension of western political control that began in 1850. By 1900, according to Chicago University historian Jo Hays, "nearly the entire land area of the globe was claimed and controlled by Europeans or their American descendants; only Ethiopia, Liberia, Turkey, Persia, China, Japan, and Siam maintained their independence. European flags flew over most of Africa, South, Southeast, and Central Asia, and all of Oceania." Europe was home to one-quarter of the world's population. Its population had almost tripled, increasing from 187 to 400 million in 100 years, and it sent at least 35 million of its own natives abroad to settle other continents. Europeans and their descendants were the substantial majority in the United States, Canada, Australia, New Zealand, Argentina, and Uruguay. European domination also entailed the "massive transplantation of other peoples from one continent to another" to meet European demands for labor, says Hays. When the slave trade died, many more non-Europeans migrated voluntarily for work, both within continents and between, spreading diseases to every continent.

When it comes to pathogens, there is nothing new under the sun, or at least very little that is truly brand new. While thirty new microbes and pathogenic agents have been identified in the last twenty years alone, including heart stoppers like Ebola and mad cow disease, the irony is that our biggest disease threats come from microbes that have been our planetary partners for many years. Our most stalwart competitors—diseases like cholera, smallpox, measles, malaria, tuberculosis, and leprosy—had reached every continent before the dawn of history. There have been an uncounted number of malaria epidemics, and we are in the seventh wave of tuberculosis epidemics and the eighth wave of cholera epidemics that first started many thousands of years ago. Together, tuberculosis and cholera have claimed many more human lives than all wars combined. On its own, smallpox claimed three times more lives than the total lost in all the wars of the twentieth century. It made its first appearance in the earliest agricultural settlements in the Levant and spread quickly through neighboring empires. Extensive smallpox lesions were found on three Egyptian mummies, including that of the pharaoh Ramses V. There were smallpox epidemics among the Hittites (1346 B.C.), and in Syracuse (595 B.C.), and Athens (490 B.C.). India, China, Korea, and Japan suffered epidemics periodically during the first six centuries of the current era, starting in 48 A.D. Smallpox was one of the three diseases that decimated Native American populations in the sixteenth century, and killed, disabled or disfigured one-tenth of the world population in the eighteenth century.

Human pathogens that have been around for a very long time become what University of Kentucky evolutionary biologist Paul Ewald calls "perpetual epidemics" because they are extraordinarily well adapted to the human species. Our basic pathogens have been around for so long that they are a permanent part of our evolutionary makeup. Many that still plague us, such as malaria and HIV, predate the separation of man and ape on the evolutionary tree. Malaria may have evolved from a simple coccidal protozoa present in our primate ancestors' bowels, and many other pathogens reside in animals just as comfortably as they do in humans. Many of our most serious pathogens crossed the species barrier a long time ago, including smallpox and tuberculosis, which crossed from cattle; malaria, HIV, and yellow fever, which crossed from primates; and measles, which crossed from dogs or deer. When HIV crossed the species barrier from monkeys, it was simply the newest example of a very old pattern.

Epidemics are not abnormal or freak events but arise predictably—and quickly—when background conditions are right. The same conditions have governed the emergence of epidemics for thousands of years. Epidemics are preceded by rapid population growth that tails into famine and malnutrition, urban crowding, poverty, and lack of sanitation and fresh water. Background conditions are so common that one scientist predicted correctly the development of a new strain of cholera from his knowledge of the biology of pathogenic agents and the conditions of population growth and poverty in south Asia. Researchers can predict the outbreak of meningitis using epidemiological data and knowledge of background conditions and of measles from information about poverty, crowding, births, and vaccination rates.

In human history, epidemics are actually signs that technological change has been so successful that population growth "overshoots" the advancement making it possible. Most major epidemics have occurred right after populations reached a peak—preplague Athens, for example, pre-Black Death Asia, Middle East, and Europe, or the Americas right before contact with Europe. At this time, the number of susceptibles—people who can catch the disease—is high. When the carrying capacity of the land is exceeded, populations are weakened by malnutrition and fall sick more easily. In the Neolithic period, new agricultural and animal husbandry techniques contributed to a remarkable period of growth, and world population rose from 15 to 150 million between 5,000 and 4,000 B.C. When the limits of carrying capacity with that technology were reached, during the next four millennia population growth slowed again. It increased gradually in Europe, interrupted by epidemics until the middle of the eighteenth century.

An epidemic is possible only if there are enough susceptible (uninfected) people to catch and pass the infection on. Although tuberculosis shows up in skeletons from 7,500 B.C., sustained epidemics of disease were rare before humans reached a certain population density. For an infection to persist, new susceptibles must be supplied through birth or migration "fast enough to feed the epidemic," British biologist Gregory Garnett says. "As an epidemic spreads through a population, the mortality and immunity it causes use up available susceptible individuals much like a fire burns up its fuel." Smallpox, endemic in India before it was eradicated in the 1970s, returned every four to eight years in epidemic strength whenever there were enough susceptible children born since the previous epidemic. For measles to persist in a group in epidemic form, mathematical modeling predicts that the group must include at least 250,000 people, which means that measles could not have persisted in human populations before the growth of large population centers. HIV builds up its susceptibles by remaining within a healthy-looking individual for seven to ten years so that person can continue to pass the disease on. While HIV jumped the species barrier at least seventy years ago, it could not rise to the epidemic levels now seen in Africa until population growth began to take off there in the 1960s.

The buildup of people not only increases the number carrying old disease agents, but increases susceptibility to new pathogens. The movement of people or goods in trade, conquest, employment, migration, or war introduces foreign pathogens, as it did with the Black Plague, syphilis and typhus in Europe. HIV is noticeably higher in urban areas and in small rural areas where people congregate once a week for markets, often no more than designated spots cleared alongside a dirt road or at a border crossing. In Africa, HIV took off first in an area bordering Lake Victoria with black market traders and major movements of Tanzanian and Ugandan troops. As people and things move from one part of the world to another, the agents of disease—diseased persons and their vectors—are brought in contact with other people who have no experience with it. Some of the world's most devastating epidemics have come from the contact of two civilizations that previously had little to do with one another. The movement of humans in conquest and trade drastically altered the population composition of entire continents, causing a complex interchange of people and diseases at many times in many places.

In the history of epidemic diseases, there are many examples of the disastrous results that occur when all of the conditioning factors intersect and contact with new disease agents occurs. The decimation of New World and Oceanic island populations, which will be described shortly, included all the ingredients, as did the conditions of the African continent after European contact. For the moment, let us take a look at the conditions preceding that classic epidemic, the Black Death in Europe. According to Hays, "by 1300 medieval Western civilization had changed almost beyond recognition from the poor, rural society that it had been four or five hundred years earlier." Cities sprang up under centralized authority, replacing local political powers of the feudal age, and there was greater security, especially for women. Women had not fared well in early medieval days, which were times of gang rule approaching anarchy, and were so outnumbered by men that scholars suspect that female infanticide was practiced. Even if it was not, the ravages of childbirth, regular dietary deficits (men were fed first), and random violence were enough to keep women's numbers relatively low. Improvements in their status and in agriculture, including the introduction of the plow, meant more calories per capita, better nutrition, extending women's life span and fertility and resulting in population growth. The cities became crowded, and trade of foodstuffs and handicrafts flourished across impressive distances.

When trade with the East opened the door to flea-infested rats infected with the bubonic plague, the formula for Black Death was complete. First, Hays says, "the European population grew prodigiously between 1000 and

1250 in part because it could shelter within a still-isolated biological environment; its growth, and that of its 'civilization,' ended that isolation." Bubonic plague, transmitted by flea bites, transformed itself into the pneumonic plague, transmitted by sneezing and coughing, and killed up to one-third of the inhabitants of any location it visited. It had already circumnavigated half of known civilization on the back of the Mongol hordes, festering in their tents, long before it hit the ports of Italy.

Crowding and lack of fresh water and sanitation in cities, coupled with an aversion to bathing, spelled a vermin-ridden population, and the opportunity for rapid spread of disease. Europe's population had weakened early in the fourteenth century, when the ceiling on food production was being reached given available technology in agriculture, expansion to marginal soils, and growing soil erosion. Food had to be transported over greater distances to cities, making them increasingly vulnerable to famine. When two seasons of heavy rainfall and cold struck in 1314 and 1315, grain stocks were exhausted, leading to a two-year famine (1315–1317) and loss of 10 percent of the population in some cities due to hunger and secondary infections like pneumonia. The birth rate was depressed and infant mortality increased. The hungry repaired to cities and monasteries in search of grain stocks, reducing agricultural output even further and breaking down the isolation of the villages.

After the plague established itself in the 1340s, it was a constant menace for over 300 years. While the Black Death from 1347 to 1350 was the most serious demographic disaster, the 1360s and 1370s saw catastrophic waves of plague, and in the poorer parts of the cities the death toll was swollen by other contagious illnesses. Waves of plague lasted from the 1300s until the 1840s in Europe, and the intervals between bouts did not lengthen until the 1400s. Repeated bouts with the plague depressed population growth until the end of the 1400s, and the plague did not disappear from north and western Europe until 1671. It continued in Spain and Germany until 1682, in Poland until 1710, and in southern France until 1721. In the western world, it was confined thereafter to Russia, which had a major outbreak of plague in Moscow in the 1770s, and to the Balkans until the 1840s. The plague left Italy but continued in the Near East and North Africa until the late 1800s. Reason for the gradual disappearance of the plague across Europe remains unresolved. Population growth had stagnated after a brief surge in the sixteenth century, but with the disappearance of the plague, it rose dramatically in the first half of the eighteenth century and was sustained in most parts of Europe until the early twentieth.

Warfare and social unrest are as perfect for encouraging the outbreak of disease in the contemporary world as they have been in any other period of history, and in this respect modern Africa resembles Europe in the Dark Ages and in the early medieval period more than it resembles the rest of the world today. Early European armies were "shakily controlled by still-impoverished governments" that could not afford to pay them. With their cannons and musketry, Hays says "the early modern mercenary army was a threat to whomever got in its way, whether friend or foe," from direct violence and as it foraged and plundered to support itself. "It remained basically unwashed, itinerant, and promiscuous, a powerful agent for the diffusion of disease," he continues, and "its incursions could completely break down the fabric of a community it attacked, including whatever provisions for health and sanitation existed." Even so, epidemics always have taken far many more lives than the wars that set them in motion and always are much more costly. While World War I casualties numbered 8.5 million deaths and 21 million wounded, the influenza epidemic carried around the world in 1918 by returning troops caused 22 million deaths and uncounted illnesses. In a sense, all epidemics are battles of a sort, battles in the war between humans and their unseen predators for control of the planet.

�֎ ✖ ✖

In western history, the most famous early reference to an epidemic is the Bible's mention of a disease that delivered Jerusalem from an Assyrian siege in 701 B.C. Attacking forces had to withdraw because they were devastated by an unidentified disease that might have been typhus. However, God was to prove himself impartial. When an army of Abyssinians (present-day Ethiopians) attacked Mecca in 570 A.D., the Koran says that God sent flocks of birds to shower stones on the invaders, spreading a pestilence among the infidels that looked suspiciously like smallpox. During the Peloponnesian War, plague raged in Athens from 431 to 423 B.C., weakening the Athenians' defenses against the Spartans and leading to a temporary truce. The population of Greece had increased to 2 million citizens and 3 million slaves; Athens alone had 50,000 citizens and 100,000 slaves, numbers that increased rapidly as peasants and shepherds took refuge from the Spartans within the city walls. By aggravating existing urban crowding, the siege facilitated the plague's spread by rodents and limited separation of sick and well. Athens lost one of its greatest leaders, Pericles, to plague, but Alcibiades was impeached when he tried to introduce legislation to control the disease. Thucydides believed that the plague hastened the demise of Greek society because it increased social and political violence while it undermined reason.

When Alexander the Great's army reached the Indus River in 326 B.C., his generals forced him to turn back because his army was ravaged by smallpox, making way for Chandragupta Maurya's reconquest of northern India in 319 B.C. Disease was a fundamental factor in the decline of the Roman Empire, ravaged by plague from 165 to 180 A.D. The plague had arrived in Rome with the return of its legionnaires from Mesopotamia. They also brought measles and smallpox to the center of the empire, which killed a quarter to a third of the population. Even Emperor Marcus Aurelius, during his campaign along the Danube, was a victim. A second wave of plague raged from 251 to 266 A.D. Commerce halted, record keeping faltered, public order was threatened, and, worst of all, the army was decimated, leaving the Romans too weak to resist barbarian attack.

Through the Dark Ages and during most of the medieval period, there was a great collision of diseases in Europe that slowed but did not cease until the twentieth century. Epidemics of tuberculosis and leprosy, related diseases, alternated with one another beginning before the modern era. Epidemic leprosy ended in Europe around 1350, but tuberculosis continued as a major killer, especially from the seventeenth to the nineteenth centuries. Scrofula and yaws, endemic in early Europe, were displaced by syphilis, which struck in the late 1400s. The great Islamic expansion from North Africa to the Iberian peninsula in the sixth to the eighth centuries brought a wave of smallpox across Spain and into France, and small outbreaks continued well into the eighteenth century. Ergotism (fungal poisoning from improperly stored wheat) struck first in the middle of the ninth century and may have returned periodically for the next 1,000 years. A long bout with bubonic plague, the type transmitted from rats to humans, occurred between 542 and 750. From 1347 to 1350, the plague returned in pneumonic form. Typhus epidemics started in 1489, when the Spanish tried to throw the Moors out of Granada. Typhus had existed in Europe before that time, but when it switched vectors from fleas to lice it became much more successful and did not disappear from Europe until right before World War I. Waves of cholera flashed through Europe beginning in the second decade of the nineteenth century. Polio is suspected as the cause of deformities depicted in many Egyptian and European texts and paintings, but was not defined as a specific disease entity until the seventeenth century. It occurred sporadically until the late eighteenth and early nineteenth century, when the first polio epidemics were reported. For some reason, it began to increase in the twentieth century until it peaked in the 1950s, when it was the fifth leading cause of death and disability in children worldwide.

This cursory history of disease in Europe makes several things very clear. For all but the privileged class, the continent was not what modern westerners would consider a very habitable place until the early nineteenth century. Europe was primarily rural until 1800, when more cities developed as the population grew. Before that, there had been some improvements in nutrition with the development of a market economy that linked rural areas with the towns, overcoming the subsistence crises that prevailed before the 1700s. Disease transmission was also reduced when the wandering mercenary armies of earlier periods were replaced in the eighteenth century by highly disciplined royal armies, which Hays describes as "less of a threat of anarchic violence and . . . less likely to diffuse typhus and syphilis through the population." There were few ways to deal with diseases or those who were infected—largely the poor underclasses, stuffed into miserable dwellings lining dense, polluted streets—until urban infrastructure was developed in the early 1800s. Europeans and Americans became more committed to clean water and sanitation starting in 1800, beginning the process of disease control in the West. When we think about disease in contemporary developing countries and why epidemics persist in those settings, Europe's experience can help us understand why basic infrastructure is necessary for disease control.

✳ ✳ ✳

The Asian mainland suffered from many of the same diseases as Europe, but at slightly different dates depending on transmission routes and relative infectiousness. In each of its major waves, bubonic and pneumonic plague showed up earlier in Asian countries than in European ones, but caused similar population losses and social change in China, India, the Caucasus, and Middle East. The plague was carried along the famous "Silk Road," the trade route connecting major capitals from east to west. The first outbreak was recorded in China in 161–162 A.D., when four out of every ten soldiers fighting on their western frontier contracted it and died. The second outbreak, from 310 to 322 A.D., killed 30 percent of the population. Public order was disrupted, and some attribute the fall of the Han dynasty and subsequent foreign invasions to the ensuing chaos. The earliest evidence of fourteenth century pneumonic plague comes from a cemetery near Lake Issyk-Kul, along the Silk Road in Central Asia. In the central steppes of Asia and the Himalayan lowlands on the border of India and China, the plague bacterium had long thrived among local marmots, ground squirrels, and gerbils. Periodic natural disasters drove these animals into villages and towns, where they made their homes in the adobe walls and thatched roofs of medieval houses. The plague recurred over wide areas of Asia from 1300 to 1550, surviving in animal reservoirs until 1855, when, Hays says, a Muslim rebellion in China's largely urbanized Yunan Province "caused two decades of internal turmoil... in which plague epidemics coincided with military massacres, famine, and considerable emigration." Plague spread along the tin and opium trade routes between Yunan and the coast and hit China's port cities hard around 1900. From the ports, it migrated to India, killing 6 million people between 1896 and 1908. It reached Madagascar in 1898. One year later it was in Honolulu, San Francisco, Egypt and Paraguay.

Major epidemics of smallpox are recorded earlier in Asia than in Europe. From the eleventh to the thirteenth centuries, the Crusades stirred population movements from Europe to Asia Minor and along the northern rim of Africa, passing smallpox back and forth in the same way the disease had traveled with seventh century Islamic invaders to Europe. Smallpox often jumped on caravans to and from Asia and into central Africa, spreading farther inland. Variolation, where a susceptible person gains immunity by getting a small dose of the smallpox virus from someone else's sores, was practiced in China as early as the eleventh century, and spread to India, Persia, and Turkey. The practice spread to Africa, and from there to the Americas in the early 1700s, when it was also introduced to Europe from Turkey. Ironically, it was in Asia and Africa that the disease hung on the longest until it was eradicated in 1977.

In the 1800s, the islands of Oceania experienced many "virgin soil" epidemics when contacts with the outside world—like the *Beagle*'s in the 1830s—became much more frequent and labor migration increased. Chinese and Melanesian laborers brought leprosy to Hawaii in the 1830s and carried the disease to New Zealand in the 1850s and to New Guinea in 1875. Measles devastated Fiji in the same year, then traveled to Vanuatu and the Solomon Islands. In 1853, 80 percent of the population of Hawaii's Oahu Island died with its first exposure to smallpox. It hit Guam in 1863 and caused similar devastation. Smallpox was carried back to Polynesia by laborers returning in the 1860s from work in Peruvian mines, and another wave of migrant laborers brought smallpox to Fiji in 1879. Syphilis was brought to Asia early in the 1500s, first hitting India, Ceylon, and Malaysia. It reached Canton by 1504, from where it spread inland and to Japan by 1569. It reached Tahiti in 1769 and Hawaii in 1779.

British railway construction opened up the Indian subcontinent, increasing the spread of diseases by religious pilgrims because it made it possible for them to travel faster, farther, and cheaper. Waves of cholera, smallpox, tuberculosis, malaria, dysentery, and diarrhea followed the movement of pilgrims and contributed to rapid and catastrophic diffusion of the plague, killing more than 8 million Indians between 1896 and 1914. Subsequent malaria and tuberculosis epidemics killed more than twice as many people, and in four months, the 1918 influenza epidemic killed even more. Death tolls from smallpox and cholera were in the millions. It was not the first time cholera hit India, but the sixth. Cholera epidemics fanned out from India to other parts of Asia, Africa, Europe, and North and South America in 1817, 1826 to 1837, 1841 to 1859, 1863 to 1875, and 1881 to 1896. The fifth and sixth, lasting from 1899 to 1923, were confined to Asia and had limited impact on Europe and the Americas due to improvements in sanitation. Because of these multiple waves, Asiatic cholera is regarded as the classic epidemic disease of the nineteenth century, as AIDS will be in the twenty-first.

❊ ❊ ❊

While the historical disease profile of Asia and Europe is very similar, varying only in the timing of epidemic waves, the picture is different in North and South America. There populations were isolated for millennia by the submersion of the Bering Land Bridge, which increased their vulnerability to new pathogens brought by the Conquistadors. Measles, typhus, smallpox, and the plague were unknown in the New World prior to Spain's first contact. However, the underlying conditions for the ensuing epidemics were similar to Asia and Europe 200 years earlier, when overpopulation was followed by famines. The Amerindians' tight kinship bonds and their fatalistic view of disease, similar to that of the Muslims of North Africa, made it impossible for them to flee for their lives when waves of disease emanated from their conquerors. They suffered the high mortality of any population that comes into contact with new diseases for the first time with devastating results. Along with forced labor and harsh treatment by their colonial masters, disease caused the extinction of the Caribbean Taino by the mid-1500s and the near extinction of other mainland groups.

A Yucatán native noted plaintively in the Maya *Book of Chilam Balam of Chumayel* that before the Spanish set foot in Mexico in the first part of the sixteenth century, "there was ... no sickness; they had no aching bones; they had then no high fever; they had then no smallpox; they had then no burning chest; they had then no abdominal pain; they had then no consumption; they had then no headache. At that time the course of humanity was orderly. The foreigners made it otherwise when they arrived here." He had a right to complain. Mexico's population was reduced from 28 million to 1 million between 1519 and 1608, and the Aztec civilization was completely destabilized, throwing the group open to European conquest. Waves of smallpox, measles, typhus, and influenza washed over the Caribbean islands of Hispaniola and Puerto Rico between the early 1500s and 1580, before arriving in Mexico in 1519. The diseases reached Peru by 1524, where the Inca surrendered to the Spanish in 1532 because they believed only gods could send crippling diseases before them as the Spanish had. Historian Alfred Crosby said "the psychological effect of epidemic disease is enormous, especially of an unknown disfiguring disease which strikes swiftly. Within a few days small-pox can transform a healthy man into a pustuled, oozing horror, whom his closest relatives can barely recognize." In some areas of Mexico, so many died that they could not be buried and were left in their houses or thrown into the wells. Annals of the Spanish empire show that between 1520 and 1600, there were fourteen epidemics in Mexico and seventeen in Peru. The Portuguese carried smallpox and influenza to Brazil beginning in the middle of the seventeenth century with the same disastrous effects.

Unique among all the world's populations, Native Americans suffered the assaults of at least four major killer diseases one after the other, amplifying the mortality that would have resulted from each one alone. Survivors were forced into slavery on colonial plantations and mines, where they were worked as beasts of burden because the Conquistadors and the church believed they had no souls and were not human. Mortality may have been higher because, Hays says, "the combination of inexplicable diseases, alien conquest, and brutal arrangement of social and economic systems con-tributed to widespread loss of will.... Ill parents may simply have given up hope and thus doomed their young children, perhaps through inadequate food, nursing, and shelter from the elements, perhaps—more drastically—through infanticide and suicide." A similar result may be seen with HIV/AIDS in Africa, especially as mortality starts to accelerate toward the middle of the first decade of the twenty-first century.

Smallpox and the other European diseases spread less rapidly in North America than in Central and South America, although Sir Francis Drake reported that when the typhus his men had brought with them from Cape Verde Islands hit the natives of Florida in 1585, "the wilde people... died verie fast." Thomas Hariot, one of the English colonists in Roanoke Island, Virginia, also reported that "within a few dayes after our departure from ever-ies such townes... people began to die very fast." The Indians in New England and Canada were hit next, in 1616, when tribes in Massachusetts were almost completely exterminated. St. Cosme, a Jesuit missionary travel-ing down the Mississippi River in 1698, reported the same devastating con-sequences of smallpox on Amerindian tribes along the river. While thirteen epidemics ravaged French Louisiana between 1698 and 1725, archaeologists believe there were earlier epidemics between 1550 and 1600. Smallpox, influenza, measles, and whooping cough were introduced to the Plains Indians and tribes in the western interior between 1774 and 1830, when Hudson Bay Company trading posts were operating. The mortality of different groups ranged from 20 to 90 percent. Smallpox was deliberately spread to Native Americans at least once, during the French and Indian War of 1763.

In the Caribbean and Central and South America, young adults seem to have suffered the most from the first waves of disease, suggesting that syphilis—which, like other sexually transmitted diseases (STDs), hits the sexually active population hardest—may have played a major role in increasing mortality. In Europe, syphilis had been as important as the plague in depressing population growth. In addition to disease, males also succumbed to colonial violence and backbreaking work in greater numbers, so women significantly outnumbered men. When the yaws Columbus's sailors introduced into Europe on their return mutated into syphilis, "the Columbian Exchange," as historian Crosby called it, was complete. The reintroduction of a more virulent strain of smallpox back into Europe in the late sixteenth and early seventeenth century, possibly from the Americas, also caused European mortality to spike again, although prior outbreaks of less severe forms had conferred some immunity.

The demographic results of European contact with Native Americans were so disastrous that colonialists, despairing at the rapid loss of plantation labor, decided to import African slaves starting in the late 1500s. Africans were especially valuable because they had developed at least a partial resistance to yellow fever, probably because of their long exposure to the disease. Yellow fever was first recorded in the Yucatán and Havana in 1648, but outbreaks were soon reported in Brazil (1686), Martinique (1690), Cadiz, Spain (1730), and later in Marseilles and Swansea, Wales. In the Philadelphia epidemic of 1793, where the fever had been carried by refuges from epidemics in Santo Domingo, Haiti, and the West Indies, 10 percent of the population died in four months. When Napoleon sent his brother-in-law, General Charles LeClerc, into Haiti to quell the rebellion of slaves led by Toussaint Louverture, yellow fever killed 27,000 of the French troops including LeClerc. As a result, Haiti gained its independence, and Napoleon abandoned his ambitions in the New World and sold the Louisiana Territory to the United States. In 1853 a yellow fever epidemic killed half the population of New Orleans, the capital of Louisiana Territory, and in 1878 it wiped out more than half of the population of Memphis, Tennessee. Finally, in 1900 Walter Reed, a U.S. Army physician, demonstrated that yellow fever could

be curtailed by controlling the breeding areas of mosquitoes, and the disease
was brought under control in many parts of the Americas.

Its position at the center of the great medieval east-west trade route exposed
Cairo to every disease epidemic that roared through in one direction or the
other. When the Black Death devastated the city in 1346, European traders
and navies were already seriously challenging its prosperity and dominance of
Asian trade routes. Egypt, which had endured sporadic outbreaks of bubonic
plague, lost one-half to three-quarters of its population to twenty recurrences
of pneumonic plague over the next 160 years. Tunisia suffered five epidemics
in the 1600s alone, resulting in what British historian John Iliffe calls "a
demographic catastrophe that ended North Africa's time of greatness," which
had begun with the Islamic expansion of the sixth century.[2] North Africa's
population stagnated from the plague, which remained there until 1835,
when Egypt's last great epidemic killed 200,000 people. Four years earlier,
Cairo had lost 150,000 in its first brush with Asiatic cholera. It swept across
the rest of North Africa, too, which never experienced enough disease-free
intervals in modern times to allow the population growth seen in Europe and
China. The end of internal warfare and the disappearance of plague after
1835 relieved some of the downward pressure on population; by 1850 Egypt
had more than 2,500 barber-vaccinators immunizing 80,000 children
against smallpox each year. Algeria experienced a similar demographic transition in the late 1800s, but in Tunisia and Morocco, efforts at modernization did not succeed until well into the twentieth century.

While North Africa shared many diseases with Europe, sub-Saharan Africa
was isolated by the Sahara and rarely had enough contact before 1800 to suffer from any of Europe's severe epidemics. The fourteenth century Black
Death spared West Africa, but other epidemics ravaged the towns of the
region, which Iliffe says had "an exceptionally hostile disease environment
[where] disease was common and debilitating, especially when compounded
by diets deficient in animal protein and vitamins." Intestinal afflictions were
common, as were parasites, largely due to the poor quality of drinking water
although the only severe cholera epidemic in the region occurred in
Senegambia in 1868 and 1869. Malaria was the biggest killer among farmers
in the area, who settled in clusters on the edges of forest clearings. Larger settlements arose in river valleys and highland areas cool enough to be mos-
quito-free. More than a tenth of the Europeans who colonized West Africa
found it a "white man's grave" in the early 1800s. Scottish explorer Mungo

Park's ill-fated 1805 expedition to the headwaters of the Niger River was reduced from forty-four members to four by malaria. As they died, expedition members were carried by their African porters, who were already adapted to the disease. At independence, a Nigerian scientist argued that a mosquito should be part of the national flag because it helped stave off European intrusion for so long.

Yaws was common in equatorial areas, and endemic syphilis was seen on the savannah, but it was a variety that was less acute than the related venereal syphilis from which the region was spared until the sixteenth century. Europeans who explored the interior reported that leprosy was common in the nineteenth century, but also in a milder form than on other continents, and only persons with the most severe cases were ostracized. Tsetse flies caused Gambian sleeping sickness, and it claimed an occasional victim (including fourteenth century King Diata II of Mali), but resistance to this disease and smallpox was high. Smallpox was milder in both East and West Africa until contact with the Europeans brought a more severe form in the eighteenth century during the slave trading period. The 1864 epidemic that killed one-quarter of the population of the Angolan capital of Luanda may have been typical of the impact of contact during the slaving period. The Portuguese in Angola reported severe famines, caused by drought, every seventy years, each one accompanied by epidemic disease that killed one-third to one-half of the population.

With so much death, Africans attached a supreme importance to child-bearing because it was essential to group survival in competitive and often violent societies. Kinship groups that fell below a minimum size were absorbed by more fertile rivals in what Iliffe calls "a process of natural selection...African obsession with reproduction later surprised anthropologists familiar with regions where nature was more benign." When trade in ivory and slaves flagged in the nineteenth century, East Africa suffered a "brutal economic discontinuity," according to Iliffe, who says nineteenth century colonial development was "only a vicious form of underdevelopment," resulting in huge population loss. Initial growth in the early 1800s was followed by steady decline after the 1850s everywhere except in Rwanda and Burundi, where growth did not flag until the 1880s. The slave trade brought brief, localized declines, but disease flourished due to famines, warfare, mobility, and clustering in large settlements for self-defense. Caravans brought small-pox; "Ganda armies seemed incapable of marching without it," says Iliffe. Epidemics of Asian and European smallpox strains had dreadful impacts, along with four cholera epidemics, and new strains of STDs.

Sub-Saharan Africa enjoyed a longer period of isolation from European contact than the Americas, and brief exposure had conferred some immunity to the diseases brought by the Europeans. Africans were resistant to malaria and yellow fever, which made them very desirable as slave labor. Although slaving caused considerable disruption in African societies, until the late 1800s Europeans had been confined to the margins of the continent. Once the continent was subdivided by five European powers in 1890, conquest began in earnest with an inevitable impact on native disease patterns. Prior to contact, Africans had achieved an adaptive balance with their disease burden. Oliver Ransford, an English "tropical doctor" who gained firsthand knowledge of disease patterns across the continent during World War I, said that "the vital years of 1885–1930 were ones of epidemiological disaster for Africa," when the "equilibrium" African peoples had established with their diseases was destroyed by "European intrusion." In Malawi, "every person . . . hosted a variety of microscopical parasites, and . . . each man, woman, and child suffered from malnutrition [and the] combination inevitably drew them into poverty and early graves. But the very presence of these sickly villagers proclaimed their descent from stock which had been able to maintain itself against the parasites that had now become their masters." After further observation, Ransford realized that "the prolonged association between their forebears and local parasites had led to a selective survival of more resistant men and women who were protected against the disease either by chance genetic qualities or by accidental possession of overlapping immunities derived from related infections. Their survival had led to a state of equilibrium between hosts and parasitic clients which allowed them to live together in mutual tolerance."

While the demographic decline was not quite on the scale experienced in the Americas, because Africa was not as densely settled, colonial intrusion was devastating and many lives were lost to warfare as well as disease. One third of Libya's population was killed during the twenty-one years of Italian conquest, and when the Germans drove Namibia's Herero into the Omaheke desert of southwest Africa, 65,000 of 80,000 total died of thirst. Military repression of the Maji Maji rebellion in Tanzania killed one-third of the population and depressed the fertility of the surviving women by 25 percent. Fighting among British, Belgians, Germans, and Portuguese in East Africa during World War I exposed more than 100,000 African soldiers and more than a million porters to extremely high death rates from disease and exhaustion. Only a few of the many would-be recruits into the King's African Rifles after the outbreak of World War II were fit for service, though army rations soon improved their health considerably.

Ecological disruption caused extensive famine during the forty-year drought that lasted from 1880 to 1920. One third of Ethiopia's population was lost between 1888 and 1892. West Africa experienced a similar crisis from 1913 to 1914, and World War I campaigns created widespread famine in East Africa, followed by a famine in French Equatorial Africa from 1918 to 1926, "owing chiefly," Iliffe says, "to excessive colonial demands for food and labor." Most famines ended in large-scale deaths from disease, because people came together looking for food and water. Millions succumbed to smallpox and sleeping sickness, which killed 90 percent of the population in affected areas of equatorial Africa. Waves of cattle plague originating in the Ethiopian famine spread through sub-Saharan Africa in the 1890s, allowing tsetse flies to move into former pastureland. Alarms were raised about the rapid spread of syphilis and gonorrhea in central and western Africa, depressing fertility and dropping birth rates to very low levels, and 20 percent of all women never were able to bear children. Sand flies proliferated across the continent, and the global plague pandemic that began in China in 1893 devastated coastal African cities. Epidemics of cholera, yellow fever and meningitis broke out, and the flu pandemic of 1918 killed 2 to 5 percent of the population. South Africa's colonies escaped most of these catastrophes, growing as fast as 2 percent per year; northern Africa experienced slow recovery. Other areas experienced some recovery starting in the late 1920s, but World War II created further setbacks. Just as Africans suspected that HIV/AIDS was created in a Central Intelligence Agency lab to exterminate them, many Africans 100 years ago thought new European diseases were magical, biological weapons created to subjugate and control them.

✕ ✕ ✕

For all the media coverage of new "epidemics" of "emerging diseases," so far none has been a major killer. Outbreaks of the Ebola virus in the Sudan, Côte d'Ivoire, Gabon, Zaire, and Uganda that occurred between 1976 and 2000 received widespread attention from the press but resulted in fewer than 1,000 deaths. The plague outbreak in India in 1994 also received such enormous media attention that it caused several billion dollars in losses to the Indian economy, although only several hundred deaths resulted.[3] By the middle of 2003, Sudden Acute Respiratory Syndrome, or SARS, had killed 800 people worldwide and World Health Organization officials predicted that future outbreaks, if they occurred, would be small and easily contained.

Far more important has been the dramatic resurgence of several old killers over the past twenty years. Diarrheal diseases, of which cholera is a major

player, account for 2,000,000 deaths each year. Epidemics of choleralike disease were first described by visitors to India in the sixteenth century, where
the disease is still endemic in the Ganges Valley, and recurred in repeated
waves for the next 300 years. Cholera's seventh pandemic began in 1961 in
Indonesia and has spread to 120 countries in Asia, Europe, and Africa, many
of which had been free of the disease for more than 100 years. It is the first
disease for which modern public health surveillance and reporting was organized, and it is still one of three internationally reportable diseases along with
plague and yellow fever. A new strain of cholera was identified in Bangladesh
in 1992 that may have originated in an upwelling of deep sea water to the
surface near the Bangladeshi coast. Scientists fear that the ocean's deep waters
act as "a kind of refrigerator" for pathogenic microbes contained in sewage
that developed and developing countries are pumping into the ocean. A variety of microbes and viruses, including polio and rotavirus, have been found
in ocean water samples taken at depths below 3,300 feet. Dysentery, caused
by the *Shigella* bacteria, caused a four-year epidemic in Central America
beginning in 1968, and has caused epidemics in Africa since 1979, usually in
impoverished areas.

In the seventeenth and eighteenth centuries, tuberculosis (TB) killed one
in five adults. It stepped up its pace in the nineteenth century, when it caused
one in three deaths and killed more people than any other epidemic disease.
It is one of the oldest diseases known to humans, found on skeletons dating
from 6,000 to 7,000 years ago, and "crossed the species divide" from domesticated cattle to humans 7,000 to 8,000 years ago. Hippocrates described it
as the most common disease of his time. Afflicting Egypt's pharaohs and
ancient Peruvian kings, TB, like HIV, is successful because it can remain
undetected in the body for many years. In 1993 the World Health
Organization declared a "global TB emergency" because the epidemic was
growing fast, and in 1995 more people died of TB than any other year in history. The disease is in its eighth epidemic resurgence and is now responsible
for 8.7 million new cases and 1,660,000 deaths each year. More than 50 million of the estimated 1.86 billion people now carrying tuberculosis have a
drug resistant strain, which accounts for 3.2 percent of new cases. Like
cholera, tuberculosis waxes and wanes following a rhythm of developing and
declining immunity in the populations it attacks.

In addition to tuberculosis and cholera, other old friends have showed up
in force. A global pandemic of meningococcal meningitis began in 1996, and
outbreaks occurred in Mali and in several other West African countries
throughout the decade along a belt that runs from Ethiopia to Senegal. In
1998 there was a major epidemic in the Sudan. At least 1.2 million cases of

bacterial meningitis occur annually, and 135,000 cases are fatal. Dengue fever, a mosquito-borne viral infection, spread widely toward the end of the twentieth century, putting 2.5 million people at risk, and there were major outbreaks in several cities, notably Bangkok. There are 50 to 100 million cases worldwide; 2.5 to 5 percent are fatal. Yellow fever epidemics occurred in Kenya and Liberia in 1992, and it is estimated that the 400-year old disease causes 200,000 cases and 30,000 deaths a year, most unreported. In the republics of the former Soviet Union, diphtheria broke out in 1995. One-quarter of the 25,000 infected people died. Hepatitus B and C account for 128,000 deaths each year.

Malaria causes 1 million or more deaths each year around the world, 75 percent of them in children. It is spreading again in Africa, with increased risk for complications and death resulting from changes in the environment, migration, breakdown in health services, and rising drug resistance. Although many have suggested that global climate changes are increasing mosquito populations and therefore malaria, "intrinsic population dynamic processes"—the natural rise and fall of the disease vectors themselves—are the best explanation of changes in disease patterns for both malaria and dengue. This is also true of cholera, tuberculosis, and yellow fever because microbes have their own rhythms of rise and decay. Malaria occurred in our hominid ancestors before they emerged as a separate species, was a well-known killer in classical Greece, and killed at least three Roman emperors—Hadrian, Vespasian, and Titus—and St. Augustine, who caught it while he was bringing Christianity to Britain. It killed millions, including James I and Oliver Cromwell, before it finally disappeared from London in 1859, when the Thames Embankment was built and drainage improved. The disease was associated with bad air—hence the name "mal-aria"—and that belief proved as tenacious as completely ineffective methods of therapy. The one exception was cinchona bark, used for centuries as a malaria treatment in Peru. When it was introduced into Europe by the Jesuits, Oliver Cromwell refused it because it was associated with the Papists. However, its success was obvious, and after the alkaloids were isolated from the bark as quinine in 1820, it was possible to give the treatment in dosages of known strength. Dutch traders grew the tree on plantations in Java and developed a profitable trade, making the drug widely available after 1854. British missionary-explorer David Livingstone became an advocate after successfully treating his children, and proved the value of the drug on his 1858 to 1864 Zambezi expedition. It was soon used by Europeans prophylactically, so they could compete with Arab travelers whose resistance to malaria had long been puzzling.

Pathogens are not as benign as many epidemiologists and biologists have led us to believe. They do not necessarily "play nice," adjusting their virulence so they do not kill off their human hosts. To the contrary, many of our perpetual plagues have developed highly sophisticated ways of hiding from us. Malaria has been successful, says biologist Ewald, in its "millions of years of battle with human and pre-human immune systems and more recently with human cultural interventions" because it is capable of a high rate of "antigen switching" that lets it hide from the human immune system. HIV/AIDS also hides from the immune system, but in a different way. Other perpetual pathogens return to animal reservoirs, like the plague; to the deep sea, like cholera; or, like anthrax, to the soil where it can survive for very long periods of time.

Only a few decades ago, experts declared that many infectious diseases were on the brink of extinction because of improved sanitation, mosquito control, global vaccination, and modern antibiotics. Flush with our early successes against them, we concluded that microbes were no competition for our big human brains. We were wrong. Epidemics had not disappeared but were flourishing in developing countries. Modern populations were growing faster than ever and population growth is still accelerating. Prior to 1950, it took the human population 3,000 generations and tens of thousands of years to double for the first time, but between 1950 and 1980 it doubled again, increasing from 2.5 billion to 5 billion, then increased to 6 billion people between 1980 and 2000. Not only is population pressure a problem for epidemic control, but it leads to migration, disorder, and chaos, the natural preconditions of disease.

As we have seen from earlier epidemics, growing populations usually signal a disease-related crash when the productive capacity of existing agricultural technology is exceeded. The proportion of the population in poverty increases, along with susceptibility to malnutrition, and efforts to provide drinking water and sanitation, still basic defenses against many infectious diseases, are undermined. "Poverty is pain," says a poor woman in Moldova. "It feels like a disease. It attacks a person not only materially, but also morally. It eats away one's dignity and drives one into total despair."[4] Polluted food and water killed 5,000 children a day in 2002. "The sewerage runs in your front door," says a poor man in Nova California, Brazil, "and when it rains the water floods your house and the waste brings rats, cockroaches, spiders, snakes, and scorpions." In the face of poverty like this, traditional public health activities are not enough. Mosquito control has been a losing battle in developing countries, and global vaccination levels are dropping, a situation that is bad for everyone because the reservoirs of infected people increase.

In the last part of the twentieth century, "largely unnoticed, the world was changing," says one disease expert. "Third World metropolises grew increasingly crowded, overwhelming sewage and water systems and providing a microbial mixing bowl for the creation of new diseases. Wars . . . spawned immense human migrations. . . . And changing patterns of temperature and rainfall allowed disease-carrying insects to extend their range . . . a menacing menagerie of bacteria and viruses skulked about, hungry for new warm-blooded hosts."[5]

In developed countries, autoimmune conditions like lupus and multiple sclerosis and degenerative diseases are becoming more common, although the world's most lethal killers are heart disease (five times as many deaths as AIDS each year) and cancer (twice as many). Up until the 1980s, scientists believed these were chronic diseases, diseases of old age that had environmental or genetic causes, and that they were noncommunicable, which means they cannot be passed from one person to another. Over the past twenty years, research has shown that more and more of these diseases have infectious causes, which may explain why more cases are occurring in younger people.

Some of our technological solutions are also turning against us. Our hospitals breed superviruses. In the United States, nocosomial infections—the kind caused by hospitals and doctors—are responsible for more deaths than AIDS, breast cancer, and a number of other modern killers to which we are more alert. About 2 million U.S. patients acquire infections in hospitals every year, and about 90,000 of them die as a result. Seventy percent of the bacteria that cause such infections are resistant to at least one of the antibiotics used to treat them, according to the Centers for Disease Control, but they spread in hospitals because staff members forget to use basic hygienic precautions. Adding antibiotics to enhance the growth of livestock also contributes to growing resistance. Even household pets harbor infections and parasites that cause major forms of physical and mental disability, including cat-scratch fever, Lyme disease, parrot fever (which affects all domestic birds), pneumocystis pneumonia, rabies, Rocky Mountain spotted fever, ringworm, roundworm, salmonellosis, strep throat (carried by domestic dogs), and toxoplasmosis. *Toxoplasma gondii*, carried by domestic cats and eliminated in their feces, is found more often in schizophrenia patients than in controls, and is a well-documented cause of human miscarriages, which is why pregnant women are advised not to keep cats. After declining throughout the twentieth century, deaths from infectious diseases rose 22 percent between 1980 and 1992 to become the number three killer in the United States, in large part due to HIV/AIDS. As changes in technology and human populations disturb our established relationships with our environment at an ever-increasing rate, we can expect that our battles with our old predators will increase in duration and frequency.

The background conditions of contemporary epidemics have changed little from those governing historical epidemics. They still include poverty—the poverty of countries unable to provide the basic infrastructure needed to control disease, and the poverty of individuals that manifests itself in their poor nutritional status, trading sex for food, migrating for work and laboring under conditions that damage their health and produce exhaustion, warfare, and social disruption. In a very fundamental way, poverty is an indisputable root cause of illness and disease. While colonialism has officially disappeared, "the global consolidation by Europeans and their descendents of wealth and decision making is a fundamental factor in perpetuation of disease," says British disease ecologist Tony McMichael. Poverty and disease are on the increase because in the past fifteen to twenty years more than 100 developing countries have suffered disastrous failures in growth and deeper and more prolonged cuts in living standards than anything experienced in the industrial countries during the Great Depression of the 1930s. Twenty percent of the world owns 80 percent of its wealth, and this disparity impoverishes the whole.

✳ ✳ ✳

According to McMichael, "the health of populations is primarily a product...of the interaction of human societies with the wider environment, its various ecosystems and other life-support processes. Within the larger scheme of things, human health and survival depends on our ability to maintain a functional ecosphere that can continue to support human biological and social needs." Responding to epidemics is one way to do that. Maintaining the environment is another. We put vast pressures on natural ecosystems, creating repeating cycles of disease. According to McMichael, "disrupted environments increase biological stresses on humans everywhere; mobility and population expansion increase their exposure to opportunistic microbes; and political or economic disruptions prevent the application of known preventions or cures." In the case of AIDS, environmental, political, and economic disruption has hamstrung prevention efforts across Africa. When we begin routinely to take the health impacts of our industries and societies into account, the outbreaks of disease that now shock us will not seem so puzzling.

Epidemics are natural forces, designed to keep the number of people and the carrying capacity of the land in balance. This is a very complex law, because carrying capacity is determined by the distribution of resources as much as the actual ratio of people to land area. If poor people in Bangladesh, for example, had enough money to build proper sewer and water systems, they would not fall prey to periodic epidemics of cholera. It could be argued that Bangladeshis are exceeding the carrying capacity of the land through overpopulation, but it also could be argued that they are deprived of sufficient resources to develop adequate technological defenses like those enjoyed by residents of New York City or Paris. For a disease to continue on as a global, perpetual epidemic, the reservoir of people carrying its microbes must be large. Unless wealthy countries do their utmost to improve conditions in poorer countries, enormous reservoirs for the maintenance of old microbes will remain. Containment, under these conditions, is impossible. Epidemics will proceed in waves as the number of people who still can be infected rises and falls, and labor migration brings in new microbes or brings old microbes to new places.

If we want to live in a world that is fundamentally safer, where epidemic diseases are less likely to break out, the connection of poverty and sustained disease reservoirs suggests that it might be in our own self-interest to redistribute income, wealth, and opportunity a little bit. If we choose not to, disease will do it for us. Every global epidemic has forcibly changed the relationship of populations in different parts of the world, redistributing resources in harsh and compelling ways. Disease has no meaning in itself; rather it "acquires significance from its human context," according to disease historian David Arnold. Disease acquires meaning "from the ways in which it infiltrates the lives of people, from the reactions it provokes, and from the manner in which it gives expression to cultural and political values." In the next chapter, we will take a look at the reactions provoked by prior epidemics to see if we can learn anything useful to apply to HIV/AIDS.

CHAPTER FIVE

Epidemic Rules, Part II: Internal Dynamics of Epidemics

When the London-based Aborigines Protection Society, an expert committee set up to protect the indigenous inhabitants of British colonies, decided to survey scientists around the world about the variety of humans in 1840, Charles Darwin took charge. He organized the world's first international ethnographic survey to learn about the origins and cultural practices of different human groups, and over the next five years, presented the findings as they came in to the annual meetings of the British Association for the Advancement of Sciences. In the course of that work, he met ethnologist James Cowles Prichard, whose *Researches into the Physical History of Man* argued that native peoples had been exterminated by colonists competing for their land and resources. Darwin had seen the phenomenon firsthand. During his voyage, he had talked with Argentina's general Juan Manuel de Rosas, who advocated extermination of the Araucanian Indians who were retaliating for loss of their land by stealing settlers' cattle and burning their ranches. A year later Rosas carried out the brutal extermination campaign he'd described to Darwin.

The idea of colonial competition also fit with Darwin's reading of Thomas Malthus's *Essay on the Principle of Population*, where he argued that human population growth would quickly outrun the productive capacity of agriculture, resulting in violent competition for food and resources. Malthus's doctrines had become central in political debates about the new English Poor Laws and the food riots stimulated by an economic depression in the early 1830s. It was Malthus's *Essay*, which also declared that many more plants and animals were born than actually could survive, that finally gave Darwin the clue he needed regarding the mechanism responsible for species change. In London's busy scientific circles, Darwin also met the social philosopher Herbert Spencer in 1838 when he joined the prestigious London Athenaeum Club. Darwin had been admitted to the Club in a block under a special ruling, along with thirty-eight other notables, including Charles Dickens. Darwin thought Spencer bright and pretentious, but Thomas Carlyle described him as "the most immeasurable ass in Christendom."

The leap to apply Darwin's theory to humans was one that everyone but Darwin was willing to make. Particularly unsettling was its adoption by Spencer's "Social Darwinists." Spencer believed that human groups were arrayed on a continuum from primitive to civilized and that human societies were approaching perfection. The public had paid little attention to Spencer's theories, but when *The Origin* was finally published in 1859, Spencer hitched his wagon to Darwin's star. It became "high fashion" to use Darwin to justify laissez-faire capitalism and oppose state control. Two months after publication of *The Origin*, Darwin moaned, "I have proved might is right and therefore that Napoleon is right, and every cheating tradesman is also right." Huxley cheered Darwin up by joking that "Spencer's idea of a tragedy was a deduction killed by a fact."

Spencer, whom Andrew Carnegie called his "Master Teacher," held that the differences between rich and poor were not the result of injustice but of biology. Yale sociologist William Graham Sumner, a proponent of Spencerian thinking, wrote that "millionaires are a product of natural selection, acting on the whole body of men to pick out those who can meet the requirement of certain work to be done."[1] Carnegie argued that competition "may be sometimes hard for the individual, [but] it is best for the race, because it ensures the survival of the fittest." To John D. Rockefeller, "the growth of a large business is merely a survival of the fittest.... The American beauty rose can be produced in the splendor and fragrance which bring cheer to its beholder only by sacrificing the early buds which grow around it. This," he concluded, "is not an evil tendency in business. It is merely the working out of a law of nature and a law of God."

Spencer's ideas became the basis for the international Eugenics Movement's aim to bring about racial purity. The U.S. Eugenics Record Office, established in 1910 by Harvard-trained biologist Charles Davenport, compiled "pedigree charts" to prove that alcoholism, criminality, insanity, poverty, and prostitution were inherited traits, and lobbied U.S. immigration to establish an office in Europe to screen the pedigree of any applicant for naturalization. Taught in secondary schools and colleges, Spencer's ideas inspired development of tests to measure fitness. The "unfit" were "often institutionalized and sometimes sterilized," while "fit" households competed in "Fitter Family Contests." Blacks, among the most "unfit" according to the laws of eugenics, were barred by "antimiscegenation" statutes from marrying whites in many states.

Spencer was a symptom of the Victorian age, when it seemed that the application of human reason could work wonders, subduing the forces of nature in the interest of human betterment. The Victorians were rightfully proud of their achievements, but they came at a cost both at home and abroad. Materials and labor from "primitive" continents were needed to feed "advancing" society in Europe. Since advancement required conquest, the benevolent provision of scientific medicine could demonstrate both their achievements and paternalistic intentions. It was a way to balance out the coercive features of colonial rule and improve the "dark masses" in white man's image. But the inexorable force of diseases proved to be more than the wonder of European medicine could handle. The curse of disease, which the Victorians viewed as a divine judgment against the primitive, trouble-some races, turned itself against the European's colonial exploitation of sub-Saharan Africa. Darwin, convinced that it was dangerous to apply his ideas about natural selection to human affairs so literally, was proved right in the end. While he knew that instinct played a role in social affairs, human social systems were so complex that tinkering with social evolution to tip the hand of nature in favor of capitalist expansion could come to no good.

Molly took one look at her friend, slumped behind the desk in her office chair, and sighed. "Robina, you look exhausted. What happened in Kasensero?" Robina straightened up and tugged at her dusty uniform. "I just can't believe how sad things are down there. On my way back this morning, one of the chiefs insisted on taking me to a house in a nearby village so I could see what was happening with my own eyes. We waited until the family was in the fields and the children were at school, and then went around to the back." She wiped the back of her hand across her forehead, pushed back from the desk, and crossed her arms across her chest. "Molly, there was a woman locked in the cow shed. She was so thin, I could see her skull underneath her skin and..." She shook her head.

Pauline sat down slowly, never taking her eyes off Robina's face. "And what, Robina? What did you see?" The tears were starting in Robina's eyes. "Well, Pauline, she'd been tied to a stake so she couldn't get away—that's what the chief said, anyhow—but this woman wasn't going anywhere.

She looked like she was dead, that's what I thought at first, but then her eyes fluttered open and when she saw us, she smiled. Just a little smile, but it was there. '*Osibyotyano nyabo*,'[2] she managed to say to me, but her lips were so dry she couldn't go on. I sent the chief for some water and went in to her. She was covered in her own filth, and the sores on her body looked like something the Devil had created himself." Robina slumped forward, covering her face with her hands.

Pauline and Molly had stopped breathing. "Why was she there?" Molly whispered. Robina sat back, wiping the tears off her cheeks. "It seems the family was afraid to touch her, or even be in the same room with her. Her diarrhea had become uncontrollable, and she had started to roam around the village looking for her lost babies. They put her in the shed so she couldn't wander, and pushed a plate of food in for her each morning. But no one would clean her or talk to her or be with her, because they were afraid to get the disease. Her children were sent to her brother's house in Masaka—that's where she came from, to work the sex trade in Kasensero when her husband threw her out after he learned he had Slim. That was two years ago. She started to decline but kept on working. God only knows how many customers she's had. She finally stopped last month because she was too weak to go on. That's when they took her children, and, after that, the chief said she lost her mind." She bit her lip.

"I stayed long enough to clean the woman's hands and face and help her drink some water." Then she looked at Molly and Pauline. "You've got to get down there, you two, as soon as you can, to wash the rest of her and get some food into her body. I'm sure she'll die in there if she's left alone any longer. How can anyone do this to a human being?"

The words to Philly's song ran through Molly's head. He had written it when he knew his death was near. "Alone and Afraid," he said. "Today it's me, tomorrow someone else." "I'll go this afternoon," she said, "after the meeting. Pauline will have too much cleaning up to do." Molly smiled over at her friend, sure that she was thinking that her own death could be alone, afraid, and without dignity, and decided that there was no sense in frightening her any more than she already was. "I'm sure that woman will revive once I get her to eat a little something. I'll talk with the family and the neighbors so that someone down there will help them. Maybe we can even get a chapter of OCBO started. It could be our second club, after Kyotera. I'm sure there's more people down there that can use some help."

Pauline looked away, and Robina closed her eyes. Desperate to change the mood, Molly reminded them about the meeting. "We've only got two hours before the Big Men arrive. We've got to make sure everything's ready before

they get here." "It's our only hope, I know. Molly, you and Pauline are ter-
rific, and I only hope we get something out of this. I can't take many more
mornings like this one. Let's get to work." Work was one of Robina's favorite
pastimes, Molly thought, and a great way to stop thinking about the wave of
death that was visiting the district. Pauline was still looking at her hands.
"Pauline," Molly said, "why don't you tell Robina how the arrangements
are going?"

When Pauline finished briefing Robina, she laughed. "The only thing you
have to do is change out of that dusty uniform into something that isn't so
'army' and write your speech. What are you going to tell them?" Robina drew
in a deep breath. "Thank you," she said. Pauline looked startled. "I mean, the
first thing I'm going to say is 'thank you' to the chiefs. They've done so much
work on this enumeration, and I want Save the Children to know it's their
work. I'll do the orphan numbers report, and then I thought I'd ask a few
of the chiefs who speak better English to talk about how Slim is affecting
their villages."

"What do the numbers look like, Robina?" Molly asked. "They're still preliminary because we have a few villages that haven't reported, but it looks like
anywhere between 12 and 24 percent of the children have lost one or both of
their parents. It's worse the closer you get to the lake. Those subcounties have
big problems ahead of them." "Phew," Pauline exhaled. "Big problems right
now, from the sound of it. That's much worse than I thought."

"Of course, not all of them are AIDS orphans, only about half. The rest
were orphaned by all the other diseases we've got down here, so the problem
will probably get a lot worse when AIDS kills more people." "What I worry
about," Molly said, "are the homes that only have children. How are we
going to look after them all?" "Well, Molly," the district administrator tapped
her pen on the desk. "That's where your OCBO comes in. People are already
pitching in. In Kasensero, they've started a community garden to feed the
children. By the way, Molly, remind me what those letters mean again?"

"Orphan Community Based Organization. But what about the reverend,
Robina? When will he speak?" Pauline muffled a laugh. "Let's save him
till last, Robina," Molly urged. "By that time, it'll be near lunch and he'll be
so hungry he won't go on forever. The way that man talks, hell would freeze
over before he was finished." "Molly," Robina interrupted, "OCBO's got day
care centers, community gardens—what else are we going to ask Save
the Children to support?" "Well, those new missionaries want to start an
orphanage," Molly started.

"Orphanage!" Robina interrupted. "If it's anything like the one I saw in
Kabula, we can just forget it! The kids have to scavenge in the neighbors'

fields to eat, and they were so flea infested, I think I'm going to send an army unit down there to help them clean up. No, we've got to get moving to support these families so the kids can stay on the land." Robina cleared her throat, thinking of the woman in Kasensero. "Whatever we do, we've got to do it now. This thing is about to overrun us. I think we can ask Save the Children to distribute food to needy families through the chiefs, but maybe we should have a way to raise money on our own so it doesn't look like we're begging all the time."

Molly brightened. "What about livestock? Couldn't we raise chicks for sale or something like that?" Robina nodded. "World Vision has that in their program, and I think it's a good idea. They also suggested giving the schools support so they could reduce their building fees. Grandparents with lots of orphans won't be able to pay, and if those kids start running around without any schooling, we'll have a real problem with security." "The credit program is working out pretty well," Molly added. "Women seem to be recovering if they get small loans to help them with their funeral costs. I think we should ask the chiefs to encourage people to limit what they spend on funerals. It's already started to happen a little now that funerals are so short, but maybe they can make it official. They're already asking people to have widows jump over the broom instead of asking their brothers-in-law for cleansing."

"Why is everything we do in this culture so tied into sex?" Pauline mused. "I know of at least twenty cases where widow cleansing ended up infecting one or the other of the partners. Well, I've got to get back to the church hall. It's eight o'clock already and I want to make sure we're on time." Molly and Pauline were almost out the door when Robina called out. "Wait a minute! How are we going to keep Wallace from giving one of his speeches?" "I've told him that the AIDS Control director will be taking care of the AIDS awareness speech, and he's intimidated enough by Dr. Okware to keep his mouth shut," Molly grinned. "Good," Robina replied. "I'll see you two at the hall."

It was only eight-thirty, but the chiefs had started to arrive. The ones from a distance had come to Kyotera the day before. "Dusty-looking bunch," Pauline muttered to Molly. "Ah, Pauline," Molly sighed. "They do the best they can. It looks like most of them are already here." She nodded at Chief Rwegarulira, from Lukunyu near the Tanzanian border. He stopped to say hello, then she and Pauline went into the church hall and started cleaning the dusty tables with a wet cloth. The dust from the road had blanketed everything as usual, so Pauline asked Florence Ngira in to help. "How's your son working out with the missionaries?" she asked Pauline. "I think it's pretty good. Mrs. Smith showed him how to make a pot roast the other day, and he showed her how to make chapattis, so I guess the blind are happily leading each other to salvation."

Florence laughed. "It was lucky they came to town when they did. My boy's selling matches and cigarettes at the taxi park." "At least he comes home with a few shillings every day," Pauline said. "And he stays out of trouble." "Well, I hope so, but some of the traders that come in are real troublemakers. Yesterday one of them asked Michael where he could find a blanket for the night." "A blanket?" Pauline was startled, then a small smile of recognition played across her face. "Did your son know what he was talking about?" she asked. "He took him to the kiosk and left him there," Florence laughed. "Either he didn't know or he did and has a better sense of humor than most twelve-year-olds." "When will he be able to go back to school?" Pauline asked. "I've almost got enough for the next term, and he's been giving me a little each day. I hope we can put it together for him because he really wants to go back." "I hope so too, Pauline replied. "He's such a bright boy."

�֎ ✖ ✖

Cristofano Ceffini, health officer in the Italian town of Prato during an especially bad recurrence of the plague in August 1630, noted in his daily record that "the epidemic started...slowly at first so that people took no notice of its gathering momentum, thinking that any day it would end. In truth, people went about their business and took little account of what was beginning to happen because they had no experience of such a catastrophe."[3] A few days later he wrote, "One learns at the cost of human life what happens when one receives from God the scourge of an epidemic without having any light or experience wherewith to guide one's conduct in so exacting a task."

Ceffini's plaintive voice still rings true today. Our inability to respond to AIDS quickly and decisively reminds us that humans can be humbled when nature takes its turn. Epidemics are history's bloodiest scythes, death for death much more powerful than war and much more meaningful in shaping human change. They are the handmaidens of conquest, deciding "both battles and the fates of European dynasties," according to historian Jo Hays. The expansionist ambitions of Napoleon were defeated twice by epidemics: in 1802, when he was defeated by yellow fever while trying to recapture Haiti after Toussaint L'Ouverture's slave rebellion and abandoned French claims to the island entirely; and in 1812, when typhus led a phalanx of diseases against his army and wiped out nearly all of them, foiling his invasion of Russia. In 1489 typhus killed 17,000 Christian soldiers in Granada, four times the number killed by Muslim armies, and set the stage for Muslim occupation. Typhus played a decisive role in the defeat of the French army besieging Naples in 1528, strengthening Spain's position in Italy and Hapsburg Germany. These losses in early modern Europe were dwarfed by contem-porary losses in the Americas, where populations were reduced by new pathogens by as much as 90 percent within a century, from 100 million to 10 million. With modern armies afflicted by HIV/AIDS, the new epidemic is just one more international security threat.

Disease, however, is only one player in the game. Epidemics are profoundly social events, in which human beings also have a starring role. Ceffini's dismay captures the frustration of humans entrusted with the burden of controlling the spread of epidemic diseases and managing their impact with insufficient resources. Plague can be cured now with antibiotics, but Ceffini had to sit by helplessly as thousands of people died. Over the ages, human responses to epidemics have become increasingly more sophisticated, but we have become effective players against disease only over the last 100 years.

Epidemic, our term for sudden and overwhelming disease events, was coined more than 2,500 years ago by the Greek physician Hippocrates, from two Greek words, *epi* meaning upon, and *demos* meaning people. This balding, bearded sage, namesake of the modern physician's Hippocratic Oath, ran the medical faculty at Cos, a Greek island off the southern coast of Turkey. Since Cos was the home to the sanctuary of Asclepius, a mythical Greek physician hero, one of history's earliest health resorts sprang up there. Hippocrates was thirty when the bubonic plague hit Athens during the Peloponnesian War in the fourth century B.C. It was the worst disaster the Greeks had ever known, and in his seven-chapter treatise called *Epidemics* he tried to make sense—and science—of it, producing history's first analysis of an epidemic disease event. *Epidemics* was one of sixty books written by the faculty at Cos to systematize existing knowledge of health and illness so that medicine could be freed from superstition and religion.

Hippocrates distinguished *epi*demics (illnesses "visiting" a people) from *en*demics (illnesses residing with a people). An epidemic is sudden, new, and affects a large number of people in a relatively short period of time. An endemic disease, on the other hand, is known, and its effects are milder but last for a longer period of time. An epidemic that has spread to more than one country is called a *pandemic, pan* meaning all in Greek. Thus, HIV/AIDS around the world is called a global pandemic, while in a single country, it is called an epidemic. The term epidemic usually involves a disease that is infectious and can be passed quickly from person to person or through insects, bad water, or animals. When an epidemic persists at a lower level, it becomes endemic.

The terms epidemic and endemic give epidemiologists—scientists trained to study disease events—a headache because there is no absolute threshold that tells us when an endemic disease becomes epidemic. Epidemics do not always involve a new disease. For example, tuberculosis and cholera can remain at subepidemic levels in a population for a long time, ebbing and flowing depending on external conditions. Use of the terms epidemic and endemic reflects how well the two costars, disease and humans, have adapted to one another. Humans can survive for a long time with endemic diseases to which they have formulated responses, but epidemic diseases emerge suddenly, affect a large number of people, and gradually taper off as a group learns to control them. As one Thai epidemiologist I worked with said, HIV/AIDS is both "epidemic" and "endemic" depending on where you live. In some countries of Africa, AIDS has become endemic after 20 years with between 20 percent and 30 percent of the population infected.

⁂

The shock of epidemics has elicited similar responses in very different historical and geographical contexts. Most of the responses we use today were shaped well before the medical profession developed even the rudiments of modern practice. Up until the late 1800s, the medical profession was as much use in dealing with epidemics as the legions of natural healers and herbalists serving the poor. Like the emetic that made Darwin's daughter vomit, physicians' cures were often fatal. When medicine adopted the germ theory of disease in the late 1800s and aligned itself with government disease control efforts, physicians became slightly more effective, but it was not until they found themselves in charge of an armamentarium of antibiotics, drugs, and surgical procedures in the 1950s that they became truly competent players in disease control. Up until that time, responses to epidemics were almost exclusively social and were relatively effective compared to medicine. Quarantine, developed by fourteenth-century public health committees to contain the plague in Europe, and sanitation engineering, beginning in the mid- to late-1800s, succeeded in separating humans from infectious microbes and in cleaning up public water and sewer systems.

While our technology has improved, one of the most important factors shaping our responses to epidemics is public attitude. As humans, our response to disease resides in the most primitive part of our brains, determining how we react to epidemics even today. Diseases and illnesses, especially when they take epidemic form, bring forth instinctual responses from our primitive consciousness. Our inherited genetic makeup tells noninfected individuals to protect themselves so they can survive and continue to propagate. Many severe diseases cause clearly visible disfiguration that evokes a "flight" response, the urge to avoid afflicted people by fleeing from them or by ostracizing, confining, or otherwise separating them from uninfected humans.

Many diseases, especially when they first enter a new population, result in severe and very visible manifestations. Smallpox causes open sores and lesions. Even after recovery, most sufferers bear visible scars. Chicken pox and measles result in sores and rashes. Leprosy eats away parts of the body, as does yaws, which can go into second and third stages and result in visible loss of bone and flesh. Scrofula produces skin blotches, as does yaws (also called pinta and bejel). Syphilis, when it first hit European populations, resulted in massive external maiming, bone breaks, opens sores, and loss of flesh on the face and head. Even the sores of syphilis and gonorrhea, hidden by clothing most of the time, are visible warnings for other human beings to avoid con-tact and contamination when sex is imminent. Tuberculosis, plague, the common cold, bronchitis, and other respiratory conditions result in racking coughs and runny noses, warning the uninfected to keep their distance.

In prehistoric and early historical times, while the mildly sick were cared for, the seriously debilitated or deformed were ostracized, ejected, stigma-tized, and isolated. Epidemics of bubonic and pneumonic plague, syphilis, and cholera are among the most memorable in history because these diseases produce the most revolting (and embarrassing) symptoms among their vic-tims, who were ostracized or quarantined. In the early-stage AIDS epidemics, before the disease becomes well known in an area, AIDS victims were isolated and stigmatized because of the disease's visible and often horrible external symptoms that rendered its sufferers easily identifiable in the last stages of their illness. When symptoms like these are bad enough, the urge to run is so strong that the urge to care must be cultivated, even among moral and reli-gious thinkers. Humanitarian responses are not natural or instinctual, but have been developed over the course of more than two millennia.

The Greek historian Thucydides's description of the plague in Athens, the earliest complete epidemic story in western literature, provided a paradigm for later writers describing epidemics, including Daniel Defoe's Black Death account, *Diary of the Plague Years*. Thucydides tells us that the Athenian "sufferers died in solitude" because their friends and relatives were too afraid to visit them; that "the dead lay as they had died, one upon another, while others hardly alive wallowed in the streets and crawled about every fountain craving for water." Victims—alive and dead—were left in their houses, in temples, in the streets, wherever they fell. Historical accounts of the Black Death when it first hit Europe speak of the same hysterical reaction. Maya historical records say that when the epidemics brought by the Spanish to Central and South America first began, the dead were not buried, but left in their houses or in the streets where they fell.

When sleeping sickness hit Uganda in 1901, patients suffering from the new disease overwhelmed Mengo Hospital, established by the medical missionaries Albert and Jack Cook in Kampala in 1897. More advanced patients were carried by their families to the forest and left to die. Albert Cook asked the chiefs to bring in a twig for everyone known to have died, and "the twigs numbered eleven thousand, and the sad little processions continued several days later," according to Oliver Ransford. Some 300,000 died of the disease in Uganda, and the Congo Free State lost one million. Sleeping sickness, limited in 1880 to small areas of Senegal, Gambia, Sierra Leone, Ivory Coast, and the Gold Coast, spread in three decades to all of east and southern Africa. The disease could wipe out whole communities, Ransford said, and "a doctor encountering an outbreak was likely to find huts filled with dying patients, together with those chained to huge logs lest they attack the few villagers brave enough to bring them scraps of food." Like AIDS, Africans blamed sleeping sickness on witchcraft. In fact, Europeans had disturbed the ecology of West Africa and the Congo Basin so much that the disease, carried by mosquitoes, quickly spread to new areas where the natives had no resistance. Its advent was sudden and swift, out of the ordinary, and fearsome. Joseph Conrad, who encountered it when he commanded a river steamer on the Congo in the early 1890s, said "the black shapes who crouched, lay, sat...in all attitudes of pain, abandonment and despair... were dying slowly, nothing but black shadows of disease and starvation, lying confusedly in the greenish gloom."

Public reactions to epidemics also depend on what people know about a disease and how it is transmitted, who its carriers are, and how they can avoid catching it. Also, as high mortality becomes more normal, as it did with the Black Death in Europe and with AIDS in Africa, public reaction to epidemic mortality becomes more matter-of-fact. Even then, however, reactions can be very negative if the disease is associated with a stigmatized social group. Among the first groups to be affected by HIV/AIDS were homosexuals, drugs users, sex workers, Haitians, and Africans, who were all socially marginalized. When HIV became more widespread, affecting people in the mainstream, such as tennis player Arthur Ashe, basketball star Magic Johnson, actor Rock Hudson, or singer Philly Lutaaya, toleration for carriers increased.

Once a disease becomes universal, says historian Paul Slack, "agreed upon communal responses may be easier to find." Historically, governments have responded best when epidemics are confined to a small group of people but are feared as an imminent risk for "ordinary people," or if they create sufficient disturbances of other social institutions, such as hospitals, and upset the prevailing social balance. Responses to epidemics of sexually transmitted diseases (STDs) have never been good because they are associated with "moral disintegration and dangerous female sexuality," says Slack. It is only when diseases threaten the wider population, especially fighting men, and become a threat to national security, as they did in World Wars I and II—or with AIDS in the twenty-first century—that they are normalized and sufferers receive the attention and treatment they need.

✵ ✵ ✵

Separating the infected from the noninfected can reduce transmission of contagious diseases because it prevents or delays passage from one person to another. Separation became institutionalized during the Black Death as quarantine and *cordon sanitaire*—when an area or an entire city is blockaded to prevent entry of infected individuals—but existed long before. The management of leprosy in Europe and Africa illustrates how these approaches changed. First mentioned as a curse in a Shinto prayer in 1250 B.C., leprosy features in Egyptian legend as the reason for the exodus of the Hebrews. In 1913 Montana State senator G. E. Willett resigned his seat when he was diagnosed with the disease. It is caused by a bacterium similar to the one that causes tuberculosis, but affects the skin, eyes, and peripheral nervous system instead of the lungs. Transmitted from person to person, probably by sneezing and coughing like tuberculosis, it can live in dust and clothing for as long as three weeks. Leprosy is one of the least contagious diseases and only 3 percent of the all humans are susceptible. The disease is not hereditary, although resistance to it may be, and since resistance is high in adults, it is believed to be transmitted during childhood, when malnutrition may increase susceptibility.

The strength of individual resistance determines if a person develops *lepromatous* leprosy, common in temperate climates, in which damage is widespread, progressive, and severe, or *tuberculoid* leprosy, a milder and more common form of the disease found in hot, humid areas of Africa, including the central African Congo rain forest, along the forested areas of the Niger, in the riverine and lakeshore areas of Zambia, the watershed of the Nile and Congo between Zaire and Sudan, the borders of Lake Victoria, southern

Tanzania, and southern Malawi. The disease develops very slowly, first becoming apparent in adolescents and young adults, and is often self-arresting. Ulcers and injuries lead to loss of body parts because a victim loses feeling in peripheral nerves. Leprosy was more common in Africa until the twentieth century, when it was displaced by tuberculosis, just as it had been earlier in Europe. In rural areas of Africa, leprosy was a major cause of poverty.

Treatment of lepers in Africa depended primarily on whether the surrounding community believed the disease to be contagious, corresponding in part to the different types of leprosy and their real relative contagiousness. Treatment also varied according to the victim's social status. In Ethiopia and Islamic societies, lepers were treated with ambivalence. In southern Sudan, where leprosy was common, even the most infected individuals freely mixed with others because no one believed that the disease was infectious. The same was true in the Kigezi area of Uganda. In Asante, lepers were sent to a sacred area near Lake Bosumtwi. Advanced cases on the Luapula were carefully isolated, but the strictest segregation occurred in the Buganda kingdoms of Uganda and in Yorubaland. Possibly as a result, colonial surveys showed less leprosy in Buganda and Yorubaland than in surrounding areas of Uganda and Nigeria, where leprosy was very common.

In West Africa's Hausaland, only more advanced sufferers were ostracized. In Mozambique, lepers lived in the community and were invited to community celebrations, but were required to bring their own eating and drinking utensils. In northern Ghana, although victims were tolerated while they were alive, elaborate precautions were taken at their burials. Changes in burial practices are common responses in epidemic times; lepers and plague victims alike could be denied church burial in medieval Europe. Changes in burial rites also have occurred in all countries with high AIDS mortality, where early AIDS victims were denied burial in sacred ground, and traditional days-long funerals have been shortened to take less time from wage and farm work.

The first colonial policies to manage leprosy were developed in South Africa. Compulsory segregation was introduced into the Cape Colony in 1892 and later into other South African colonies. While some degree of segregation had been traditional, sufferers viewed their forced removal from their villages and confinement in a special settlement for life as living death because it often was. Leprosaria were remote, had no medical help, no drugs, and were poorly served, so their inmates made frequent efforts to escape. The superintendent of the Pretoria Leper Asylum requested ten-foot fences of barbed wire, watchtowers, and warning bells. By 1920 the total number of lepers in South Africa had declined to 2,248, but the cost of control was as much as all other diseases combined. Ironically, confinement was not entirely responsible for the disease's decline. Rapid urbanization during the period was spreading tuberculosis, which confers immunity to leprosy. In Basutoland (present-day Lesotho), where confinement was also compulsory but not well policed, at independence in 1966 leprosy was uncommonly high but there was little tuberculosis.

In German East Africa, segregation was compulsory, but the 4,000 lepers in the colony's forty-seven authorized leprosaria were only a small a fraction of the total because government authorities recognized "that they could neither cure the patients nor in practice hold them against their will," according to British historian John Iliffe. At the turn of the twentieth century, the British tried to forcibly remove lepers from the West African kingdom of Igboland to confinement camps, but the policy collapsed because it was too costly and incited local resistance. In northern Nigeria, the British provided sanctuaries for more than 1,000 advanced cases, and several neighboring Hausa emirates provided similar care. In other African colonies, care was left to missionaries, who provided "sanctuaries for a tiny minority of sufferers," Iliffe reports.

It was not until 1925 that Sir Leonard Rogers, a physician working in India, convinced the British colonial administration to try treatment with chaulmoogra, a derivative of hydnocarpus tree oil used by physicians in India for many decades, in Africa. Dr. A. B. Macdonald of the Church of Scotland mission hospital in Nigeria began injections in 1926, and as always in Africa, real help attracted unexpected numbers. Within six months Macdonald had a settlement of 400 patients, supported both by the British and native administration, that became a model for the rest of Africa. Effective treatment drew lepers who had previously hidden themselves, and the colonial administration realized the disease afflicted many more Africans than had been believed, some 200,000 in Nigeria in 1936 alone. Treatment was provided in Togo, Nyasaland, Uganda, Tanzania, Zanzibar, and Kenya, which still had 35,000 active cases in 1950. In southwestern Sudan, 5,000 sufferers were gathered into three huge camps for treatment between 1928 and 1930, 40 percent of whom were successfully treated and released by 1935. French mission hospitals also provided the cure and created elaborate settlements where educated lepers with less advanced cases helped treat others. Leprosy workers were the humanitarian heroes of their time because some contracted the disease, but regular care usually was provided by African assistants, nurses, and dispensers.

In the 1950s, governments took over treatment from the mission hospitals, curing the disease with antibiotics instead of providing long-term charity or salvation. New admissions peaked in the early to mid-1950s, but leprosaria continued to operate through the 1980s to care for advanced cases or sufferers who were ostracized or destitute. Leprosy still afflicts 20 million people in eighty-seven countries today, only 20 percent of whom have access to treatment. India and Brazil have the highest modern prevalence, but there are 200 new cases each year in the United States. Treatment with antibiotics is effective, but a vaccine has not yet been developed because the bacterium cannot be cultivated in a lab. Since almost 97 percent of all humans are naturally immune, it is probably a very ancient disease. Leprosy's only other known natural reservoir besides humans is the armadillo.

⌘ ⌘ ⌘

Leprosy was rampant in medieval Europe, its growth exacerbated by a general lack of bathing and the miserable living conditions of the poor, forced into close and prolonged contact with one another in crowded, leaky huts. European skeletons from the fourth and fifth centuries show extensive damage from the disease. While leprosy was common, its exact prevalence, morbidity, and mortality are difficult to establish because early European and medieval population statistics are poor and lepers were quarantined and stigmatized throughout Europe. Tuberculosis, plague, and other diseases probably caused more deaths even when leprosy was at its height in the twelfth and thirteenth centuries.

The first laws controlling leprosy date from eighth-century Carolingian France, but it was not until rapid population growth and increased crowding in the eleventh to thirteenth centuries increased spread that "comment about leprosy, consciousness of it, and vigorous response to it peaked," according to Hays. Lepers were confined to leprosaria after being administered last rights, covered with cemetery dirt, pronounced dead, and prohibited by a priest from entering churches, markets, mills, or taverns. Lepers were forbidden to go barefoot, wash in a public water source or stream, live with any woman "other than your own," or touch a child, and were ordered to avoid narrow lanes and place themselves downwind of anyone brave enough to initiate a conversation. After dressing in a distinct costume, they were led to their own community, or leprosarium, outside the town walls. Legally dead, lepers could lose ownership of their property and were refused the right to make contracts or inherit property. If uninfected, the spouse could be declared a widow or widower and eventually remarry.

Lepers were viewed with repugnance until 1206, when St. Francis of Assisi, having renounced his father's fortune, knelt down and gave an embrace, a bit of comfort, and a few sympathetic words to a leper he met on the road. He restored a family villa where he nursed lepers. His acts of compassion for lepers, which included begging for their food, feeding them, and washing their sores, not only developed his own grace, but prompted a complete reversal in public attitudes toward lepers. People came to believe that lepers were chosen by God to suffer for all mankind, and they were rewarded with alms from the repentant. In some towns they were allowed to wander the streets, wearing bells to warn others of their approach.

All the same, the leper was clearly sinful, commonly accused of lechery: "lepers were schemers and deceivers who cuckolded the faithful, and they burned with overpowering sexual urges," according to Hays. A campaign against heresies of all types began, including mass repression of homosexuality. In the twelfth century, the Archbishop of Canterbury, St. Anselm, asked that the punishment be moderate because "this sin has been so public that hardly anyone has blushed for it." Up to that time, the practice—more or less accepted in about two-thirds of all human societies at one time or another— had been tolerated by the Catholic Church, and homosexuality was widespread in monasteries, extolled by St. Aelred of Rivaulx as a "way of discovering divine love." Richard the Lionheart was among many pious Crusaders whose sexual preference for men was well known. By 1260 the tide had turned, and penance was no longer thought to be enough. France initiated the persecution, requiring amputation of the testicles for the first offense, of the penis for the second, and death by burning for the third.

By the fourteenth century, physicians abandoned the association of leprosy with "hot" blood, thinking instead that its cause was too much bile, leading to depression, irritability, and melancholy. Whether sanguine or bilious, a leper was, by that time, clearly understood to be contagious, although this conclusion had been reached in the face of contrary evidence that many lepers did not pass the disease to their spouses. The clue about contagiousness came from a recovered Hippocratic text that mentioned that the disease could be passed from a leprous mother to a nursing child. Lepers were no longer expelled from leprosaria for misconduct, and leprosaria, formerly places for spiritual contemplation, reconnection, and repair, became places for strict quarantine. Although Arab authorities already knew the disease was contagious, lepers were not quarantined in Muslim societies because they viewed the disease as Allah's will and took no action to avoid it. Christians, on the other hand, were directed by their faith to isolate lepers because they had been stigmatized by God.

By 1100 the western world was rediscovering Greek and Roman medical texts, partly through the work of Arab scholars like al-Rhazes and Avicenna, both of whom "deeply influenced Western medieval thought," according to historian Jo Hays. Naturalistic explanations of disease made slow headway against divine will among Christian thinkers until twelfth century European intellectuals rediscovered the anatomical and etiological theories of Galen. Newly evolving universities combined classical thought with Christian ideology, and a new class of medical professional, the physician, emerged. But while theory of disease was changing rapidly, it had relatively little effect on mortality or health. Formally trained physicians who might employ Galen's theories were found only in larger towns, accessible only to the upper classes. While the intellectual tradition was growing, most people in medieval Europe still relied on divine intervention and an assortment of herbal and traditional healers.

The disappearance of leprosy outside of Scandinavia was initially attributed to the rise of the plague in the mid-fourteenth century. Lepers enjoyed some immunity to plague, but plague-related economic declines also shrank their support systems and increased their mortality. Several other factors played a role. Yaws, common during the medieval period, was probably misdiagnosed as leprosy, which declined when the two conditions were distinguished. Tuberculosis can cause scrofula, resulting in dark, discolored, putrid blotches on the face and neck that also might have been confused with leprosy. Finally, leprosy and tuberculosis are related, confer cross-immunity, and fluctuate with population density. Following the decline of Rome, leprosy displaced tuberculosis in the rural early Middle Ages, but as Europe's population increased between 1000 and 1300 A.D., tuberculosis spread rapidly in urban crowds, displacing leprosy.

✳ ✳ ✳

As changing attitudes toward leprosy in Europe show, religious opinion was a critical ingredient in shaping European thought about illness. Belief that epidemics, death, and disease are manifestations of divine judgment is common all over the world. The fear created by disfiguring diseases is so profound that even when they can be explained by science, they also are connected to beliefs about the supernatural. To early Christians, illness was a sign of the sufferer's spiritual decay, a mark made by God to help others isolate and punish the victim. The connection between disease and individual sexual habits that began with leprosy was reaffirmed by Calvinism, which arose at the same time as syphilis was spreading in Europe in the early 1500s. At the height of the plague, the Venetian Senate declared that "God is accustomed to show us the scourge of his wrath, to recall us to good and to the better way of his service." In the early days of HIV/AIDS in Africa, witches were identified and punished. Even after the disease became so common that everyone knew a carrier, superstition played a major role in explaining who got it and who did not.

Early Christian beliefs grew out of earlier Jewish traditions, which in turn shared a supernatural view of illness and disease with surrounding Mesopotamian cultures. The Jews believed God's wrath also could be directed at an entire people, expanding on the Middle Eastern belief that it was reserved for individual miscreants. God's wrath was a reasonable explanation for widespread epidemics and natural disasters that could not be explained any other way. The diseased were (possibly quite literally) the "unclean," so sufferers of skin diseases and other obvious spiritual blemishes were banished from the community for the protection of the godly, the healthy, the good, God's chosen, the unblemished. These beliefs persisted through the Renaissance, until a crude understanding of contagion emerged when Greek texts were recovered by Muslim physicians.

To the Greeks, health signified individual spiritual and moral balance. Disease occurred when balance was lost. This belief, the Greeks' anatomical studies, and their accumulated knowledge of herbal lore and healing plants from surrounding cultures—the *materia medica* of early medicine—was lost to medieval Europe with the spread of Christianity. Healing practices that involved cleansing and bathing also were lost when the sophisticated indoor plumbing systems, reservoirs, and piping of Greek and Roman civilizations were forgotten. Early Christians gave little credence to the bathing, herbal remedies, and cleanliness emphasized by other religions, preferring exorcism to exfoliation.

When Christianity first developed, plagues were rampant throughout the Roman world, hastening the empire's decline. The first Christians saw that Greek and Roman healing traditions were powerless in the face of the plague. Since Christ had been a healer, however, caring for the dying was an important spiritual obligation, and the healing power of divine touch was a sign of kingly legitimacy and power. By the third and fourth centuries, Christian thinkers advocated a synthesis of their spiritual healing techniques with classical medicine, but by then the anatomical and herbal texts of Hippocrates and Galen had been lost. Although the Arabs maintained the Greek medical tradition and diffused it during their sweeping conquest of Egypt, North Africa, Spain, Palestine, and Syria in the seventh and eighth centuries, its association with infidels caused its virtual disappearance from Europe until after 1100.

The guilt and fear that played such a major role in shaping European reaction to the plague was not universal. In Egypt, mortality from the plague in 1348 was as high as in Europe, but social strain and hysteria were minimal. In Europe, the Apocalypse seemed to be at hand, but Muslims bowed serenely to God's will. Muslim attitudes toward the plague were shaped by intense theological discussion during the Islamic expansion from the Middle East across Europe and Asia, which coincided with the middle years of the 541 to 749 plague pandemic. Attitudes toward disease were shaped along with other aspects of theology, where approaches to epidemics played a relatively minor role.

Muslims, like many other medieval Near East peoples, had believed for more than a millennium that epidemics were caused by *afreets*, demons and spirits who spread pestilence among mankind using various weapons. While *jinns* (good spirits) and *shayatin* (bad spirits) were responsible for an individual's luck, pre-Islamic Arabs also knew that *adwa*, or contagion, was responsible for the spread of disease among their camel herds and leprosy among people. The Qur'an acknowledged the existence of demons, but in the newly developing religion, the all-powerful and all-knowing God had to be placed higher than *afreets*. In the growing Muslim theology, devastating powers could not be acceded to minor spirits, and disease causation could not be due to the capricious infection of individuals regardless of their good or evil deeds. Salvation from a horrible death could not depend purely on chance or access to a means of flight. Since the faithful and the infidel were equally afflicted by plague, a new tradition arose whereby a good Muslim who died from the plague or certain other diseases would not have to wait for Judgment Day but would proceed directly to Paradise. Death was martyrdom, the plague a heaven-sent "gift" without the stigma of wrongdoing. Acceptance and acquiescence were marks of the truly faithful.

�֍ �֍ ✖

To Europeans buffeted by the hardships of the preceding one hundred years, the Black Plague was just another version of divine wrath, lurking as a dark spiritual force in the people's imagination. "We see the death coming into our midst like black smoke, a rootless phantom which has no mercy," wrote Welsh poet Jeuan Gethin in March 1349. When it first hit in 1347, the plague overwhelmed organized medicine, already weakened by its failure to respond to the challenge of leprosy. With no systematic theories of cause and treatment, formal medicine had little authority over the competing alternatives, bodies of folk healing and herbal remedies shaped by long periods of trial and error. They were effective with known diseases but of little use with new ones, especially one that hit with the force of pneumonic plague. Since Europeans knew that contagion might play a role in transmission, they closed their ports to ships with plague victims aboard, tossed the dead, dying, and ill over town walls, and denied entry to refugees from neighboring plague-infested communities. Blame was cast on lepers and Jews, who were slaughtered in Frankfurt, Mainz, Cologne, and Brussels by armies of Flagellants, who also directed their anticlerical fury at civil authorities and wealthy elites. Bad airs, or miasmas, also were suspected of transmitting the disease, so Pope Clement VI barricaded himself in his palace, surrounded by fires to purify the atmosphere. Even domestic dogs and cats, blamed for the spread of the disease, were massacred, giving guilty rats an additional advantage.

While almost all communities ground to a halt for a few months—business ceased, imports died, industry closed, and agriculture was neglected—some rebounded quickly and others devolved into anarchy. The governments of Siena, Perpignan, Pistoia, and Orvieto remained sufficiently organized to help their cities' inhabitants write wills and settle estates, recruit new workers to replace the deceased, and organize taxation and finance to maintain their armies and provide relief to hard-hit villages. Despite the loss of public managers in the person of bailiffs and agents, cities in the English Midlands restored their legal routine following several months of hysteria. Additional waves of the plague rolled over Europe, disrupting communities that had sustained themselves through earlier strikes, and the tensions mounting from rapid fluctuations in power eventually erupted. The plague became a catalyst that set in motion or accelerated larger social and economic events, and the Renaissance, Protestant Reformation, and Age of Exploration were all played out on a plague-infected stage.

European views changed as the plague continued for three centuries and understanding of the role of contagion grew. As early as 1348, northern Italian cities took sterner measures to reduce infection, and remarkably intrusive systems of public health developed. City governments established public health committees that became permanent boards as repeated waves of the plague washed over Italy. In 1486 three Venetian noblemen, elected annually, began supervising measures to control the plague within Venice and in subordinate towns and villages. Florence followed suit in 1527. Milan's duke appointed a health commissioner in 1437, replaced by a board in 1534. It was the Venetian board that introduced the idea of quarantine—from the Italian *quarante die*, or forty days—the length of time which suspected carriers were isolated to determine their status.

The boards were administrative, not medical, although Milan's board included two physicians. Initially they inspected everything that could possibly relate to bad air, but as the contagion theory took hold, they began regulating church services, meetings, schools, and marketplaces, closed and fumigated infected houses, seized private property for use as "pest houses" for the infected and convalescent homes for survivors, and collected statistics on the infected. They inspected cross-border trade and travelers, erected *cordon sanitaire* around infected areas, and issued and inspected health passes. They separated infected family members, whose banishment to the pest house was a virtual death sentence, and also could refuse them a church burial. Their sweeping powers led to tax increases and to open conflict with civil authorities, the clergy, and the business community, because a quarantine could cripple a city's trade and industry. Publicity about plague could dampen an entire city's commerce, and boards often struggled to resolve the interests of disease control and business. Their conflicts with physicians, who belittled their judgments, led to riots, widespread corruption, and bribery. Health officers took bribes in money and property and extorted sexual favors.

Epidemic policing caused many to question the limits of state authority exercised in the name of public good. In early modern Italian cities, public health authorities clearly curtailed individual freedoms and interfered with social traditions. Recognizing the vital need for these boards, Milan's and Florence's city governments refused to recapitulate to the demands of commercial interests, and gave their boards broader powers. They decreed that an attack on their officers was a major crime and gave them the enforcement powers of arrest and torture. In this highly charged atmosphere, Hays says, "the health measures themselves were sometimes the products of political forces, [not solely] reactions to the pressures of epidemic disease" and state actions against disease "occurred in the context of state economic and social manipulation."

In Florence, after studying the public health committee's data, city fathers concluded that "the poor (and especially their children) were the most likely carriers and hence in most need of control," Hays continues. Wealthy elites found this conclusion comforting because uprisings were becoming more frequent. Plague was mixing with other diseases common among the poor, such as tuberculosis, because of their marginal living conditions, compounding the threat of contagious disease. Although in Italy disease was viewed as a social problem associated with poverty and disorder, its roots were believed to lie in individual sin, so religious and secular opinion aligned in favoring isolating the victims in pest houses and placing *cordons sanitaire* around the poor areas of the city. In the eighteenth and nineteenth centuries, these regulations sparked rebellions among the poor, and when quarantine of the poor was enforced in response to cholera outbreaks in the nineteenth century, riots broke out in many European countries.

✖   ✖   ✖

Epidemics aggravate the tendency to channel resentment by scapegoating groups of people who are different, deviant, or outsiders. Communities identified witches or other scapegoats—often, in Europe, the Jews. But vagrants, seasonal migrants, war refugees, and prostitutes were all, at various times, blamed for spreading the plague and were expelled from their communities or imprisoned with very little provocation. The poor were also outsiders because they threatened established systems of wealth accumulation in society, and their survival required behavior on the edges of social ideals. With the rise of Calvinism in Europe, the poor were understood as targets of God's wrath, incorrigibly ignorant of proper social behavior and cleanliness. In the preplague days of 1630, Venice, like other Italian cities, passed two decrees to clear beggars out of the city's sacred quarters in order to propitiate God. Since the improvident behavior of the poor—their fecundity, their "failure to follow the example of the rich by restricting marriages"—was thought to be responsible for the plague, disease was seen as a divine instrument that would remove the surplus population. At the same time that the plague drove the poor to desperate measures to avoid starvation, plague deaths acted as a control. Decimated and enfeebled by disease, the poor became less of a threat to the wealthy elites.

The plague eventually killed 30 percent of Venice's inhabitants, although the Senate tried to protect the city by inspecting the quality of food, reducing the movement of infected goods, separating the sick and the uninfected, and providing oil, fresh water, and firewood to the poor. By 1540 the Venetian board of health's powers included poor relief, suppression of begging, and control of prostitution. Helping the poor was both a way to placate God and a practical way to contain the plague. Meeting their needs was a requisite for political survival in cities where the working poor and indigent formed at least two-thirds of the population, but as the plague persisted, employment disappeared when wealthy business owners fled. Facing destitution, the poor were abandoned to the whims of the plague because they could not afford to leave the city. Panicked country dwellers added their desperation to the urban masses, coming to the city frantic for bread and charity. City fathers searched for ways to "decentralize" charity to avert these invasions, but as the plague got worse, there were few resources to spare. In 1630 some 44 percent of the Florentine population needed public relief. Although authorities knew that the daily living conditions of the poor included contact with polluted water, damp and crowded living quarters, and the musty-smelling silkworms that provided their employment, they were never inspired to address housing conditions in a systematic way to forestall the next disaster. Hays thinks that "the failure of the plague to make a more lasting impact on social policies [was because] it also controlled the dimensions of poverty."

The poor who survived benefited in the long run because higher death rates created labor shortages, higher wages, and eventually freed western European peasantry from the oppressive bonds of feudal agriculture. The plague broke the back of feudalism in western Europe and made space for the rise of the middle class. It modified the relationships of landed elites, peasants, and workers, ending the manorial system and increasing the importance of towns and central political authority. In eastern Europe, the landlords' position had been strengthened, and they tightened their bonds on serfs. Construction workers who survived had more work than they could handle and began using designs that took less time to build, so that a simpler architectural style replaced the ornate Gothic common before the plague. Thousands of villages were abandoned, and in the towns, the epidemic caused tremendous short-term disruption in markets, transportation, banking, and production, leading to a decline in urban crafts. But productivity and prices soon recovered, and the demand for fancy goods and foodstuffs gradually revived as survivors of the Black Death reacted with conspicuous consumption.

For some, the bonds on social behavior were loosened by the apparent inevitability of death, but others pursued strict morality with renewed vigor. Hays says the plague "touched off long-simmering resentments against the Church," which condemned new, informal religious movements that developed to fill the vacuum created by plague deaths among the clergy. Better than half the clergy died because their cloistered living arrangements fostered rapid disease spread. Formerly thriving monasteries were decimated and abandoned. Many clergy fled, and greedy priests abandoned their poor parishes to go to cities to sing requiem masses for the rich. Laypeople turned away from religion, disillusioned because it had failed to prevent the epidemic. The Flagellant movement was born, penitents who paraded through Europe's cities, whipping themselves with leather thongs tipped with metal spikes to atone for their sins. Especially strong in Germany, it was banned by Pope Clement VI, who saw in it the basis for widespread revolt against church control. The pope also condemned unfair treatment of Jews and forbade any Christian from harming them, but Jews were repeatedly attacked and tortured for allegedly poisoning the drinking water. For generations afterward, religious thinking focused on ideas of the Apocalypse, and dissatisfaction opened the way for the Reformation.

Medicine also lost face. Many physicians fled plague-infested cities—as Galen had from Rome during the second century plague, Sydenham from

London in the seventeenth century, and physicians in Philadelphia and New York during eighteenth century yellow fever outbreaks. They charged higher fees or refused to visit acutely ill patients, negotiating with the state so that surgeons, with a lower status, had to shout the sex and condition of the patient to the physician from an open window. When a doctor denied care to plague victims in Rome in 1656, the cardinal in charge of the health board arrested him and made him serve in a plague hospital. Physicians were forbidden to leave some cities, were seduced into contracts with others by the promise of citizenship and high wages, and were accompanied by a guardian to ensure they had no contact with the uninfected. With the death of scholars and professors, many colleges closed, and knowledge of classical languages, long the hallmark of higher education, declined. More importance was attached to the native languages of Europe and nationalism spreading across the continent. With the loss of old authority, people became more concerned with individualism, materialism, and worldliness. Pope Clement despaired: "The father did not visit the son nor the son his father. Charity was dead and hope crushed."

"Oh happy people of the future," Petrarch wrote, "who have not known these miseries and perchance will class our testimony with the fables."

※ ※ ※

The waves of plague that raged through Europe from 1347 to 1650 slowed and suddenly came to an end in 1650, but the public health measures they provoked had become routine. Long-term efforts to help the poor flagged when the disease died down. The nobility's management of the plague had caused widely different death rates among rich and poor. The accusations and counteraccusations it provoked broadened political awareness in the same way AIDS is raising awareness among the poor in developing countries today. The spread of cholera across nineteenth century Europe provoked similar responses. It was a disease of the poor that offended upper-class Victorian sensibilities, an invader from the East that challenged European assumptions of cultural and biological superiority. Even the most civilized people were vulnerable to a disease associated with Oriental backwardness. Cholera shook the confidence of a bourgeois society that thought it was the epitome of progress and civilization, a confidence that only could be regained by blaming the uncivilized, poverty-stricken masses. For their part, the poor stopped blaming witches, Jews, and other scapegoats as they realized that the spread of the disease among them was a result of exploitation. They suspected that cholera was deliberately spread by the rich to reduce their numbers, and in

Prussia, the poor believed that doctors were paid as much as three thalers for every cholera death they reported to the king.

Caused by polluted drinking water, cholera epidemics hit the poor disproportionately, and the difference in its impact on social classes was as plain as the difference in their living conditions. In 1892 the great biologist Robert Koch described Hamburg's inner city as "Asiatic." One outraged Hamburg bourgeois exclaimed, "Never had I... realized what poverty concealed itself behind the proud and resplendent buildings of the great city, how dreadful was the chasm that separated the frontage and the houses behind. Those were not even people of the same era, the same land, the same race." Visitors from more "civilized" European countries had great fun tsk-tsking Hamburg's conditions. A *London Times* correspondent said it was "the dirtiest town I had ever seen on this side of the Mediterranean... tall houses excluding light and air from the narrow roadways... walls and pavements greasy, dingy, and forbidding. And then those dreadful canals. You could almost fancy the cholera rising in visible shape from the four and stagnant water bordered by black slime." The disease hit the poor inhabitants of the canal district hard, and they were rewarded with slum clearance. Clean-up efforts put the state budget into a ditch. When a major tax increase was proposed, the Senate cut the scale and scope of all public health projects, leaving conditions pretty much as they were before the epidemic.

Biologically, the impact of cholera on poor people is much worse because malnutrition reduces stomach acid production, the body's natural defense against the disease. Cholera epidemics coincided with years of political unrest in Britain (1832), France (1848), and Germany (1866), where reckless failure to address the hygienic needs and wars of adventure wracked society, spreading the disease and interfering with farming. Both 1847 and 1848 were famine years in central Europe, and starvation pushed rural people out of their homes to look for relief in the towns. Waves of unrest swept the continent; riots, massacres, and destruction of property broke out in Russia, Germany, Britain, and Scotland because the poor believed the rich were poisoning their water supplies. In Hungary, after more than 1,000 people died of cholera in less than four months in the summer of 1831, nobles were murdered and their castles destroyed. Cholera challenged trust and cooperation, bringing latent social antagonisms to the surface.

Until the cause of cholera was discovered, the public health measures that were employed to contain it, developed in response to the plague, only worsened its spread. During the seventeenth and eighteenth centuries, state power had been consolidated to a much higher degree than during the Black Death, so public health policing could be carried out more efficiently and with much less local participation. When quarantine and *cordon sanitaire* reduced urban food supplies and disrupted livelihoods, popular resistance grew. Public suspicion was aroused when inexplicable outbreaks of mass mortality coincided with the sudden arrival of government officials, troops, and medical officers. In Great Britain, where the state was less aggressive, physicians were attacked by crowds who believed they were killing off the poor to obtain corpses for anatomy courses. That idea was plausible, given contemporary medical practice. In 1828, a year after Darwin left Edinburgh, William Burke and William Hare killed at least sixteen people in the city's crowded poor section to supply the medical school with cadavers. In France, the wealthy were blamed for poisoning the water supply, and hospitals were reviled as places of medical experimentation on the poor. Even reformers and radicals became afraid of the poor, convinced that cholera had been spread by the state to discredit the reforms being promulgated to help them.

Historian Jo Hays says that Europe's plague and cholera epidemics demonstrate that "the poor get not only the blame, but also the disease." Even tuberculosis, long romanticized as a disease of upper class aesthetes, poets, and the artistically gifted in the nineteenth century, was a disease that inflicted horrible morbidity and mortality on the poor. Disease sharpens class and economic differences within societies. It also aggravates the normal disdain upper classes have for the lower, and the disdain held by longtime settlers for immigrants, even when their labor is essential to upper-class well-being. The poor were viewed at best as inconvenient, at worst as harbingers or vectors of disease, dangerous to the upper classes. Even among the enlightened, epidemic outbreaks are always associated with moral failing, with God's judgment and His disdain for poverty, filth, and sloth. And while their condition results from denial of their basic human rights, poor people do form a permanent reservoir of disease within many societies.

Many European governments relaxed their disease control efforts after the 1830s because of protests and pressure from merchants, traders, and manufacturers. Commercial interests are always at odds with disease control measures, which require expenditures of public resources and tax dollars, the redistribution of wealth for the provision of common services such as sanitation, food, and other forms of social security. Physicians supported government decisions to withdraw public health measures, arguing that mass hysteria did little to reduce the spread of the disease. By 1848 the weight of medical opinion was against the idea of contagion—not fully understood until the late 1800s—reinforcing government decisions to take no action. Russia, which refused to relax public health restraints while making no effort to improve the conditions of the poor, was the only government that continued to experience mass unrest. Cholera and plague persisted in eastern Europe and Russia through the late 1880s. Robert Koch's discovery of the bacillus responsible for cholera in 1884 changed the attitudes of European governments. Massive prevention campaigns were instituted, including public education campaigns to improve personal hygiene, disinfection, and quarantine. Professional police forces, created after the revolutions of 1848, quickly swept aside any resistance to public health policy.

The history of yellow fever in the United States also illustrates the conflict of contagion and commerce. Yellow fever hit Philadelphia in August of 1793, then the nation's capital with a population of 55,000, making it one of the largest English-speaking cities in the world outside London. The disease arrived with refugees from Haiti, and by October 5,000 were dead and 20,000 had fled the miasma, or bad air, of the city. Yellow fever had devastated Native Americans and new arrivals in Philadelphia, New Orleans, and Charleston during the early years of American settlement. With yellow fever raging, Philadelphia's physicians were divided about its cause, and their deliberations were politicized when Alexander Hamilton recovered from an attack under the care of a physician who advocated an alternative regimen to the one proposed by the city's medical establishment. Merchants, anxious that the theory of miasma be overturned so that Philadelphia would not be condemned by the rest of the world, pushed the state government to act on the contagion theory and quarantine incoming goods and people. Other American cities responded with a boycott. Halfhearted attempts were made to clean up the garbage and the air, but as the epidemic worsened, services collapsed and the federal and state governments closed down. The mayor heroically assembled an *ad hoc* citizens' committee that opened an isolation hospital and an orphanage, raised money for emergency responses, provided care for the sick, and buried the dead, similar to the city committees formed in the Italian Renaissance. Before the epidemic receded with cooler weather, 15 percent of the city's population had died. In its wake, Philadelphia lost its position as the U.S. capital because survivors feared further outbreaks of the fever, and it declined as a great seaport, opening the way for the rise of New York.

❊ ❊ ❊

Physicians had no edge over competing healers until the late 1700s, when several developments strengthened their position. Beginning in France in 1803, government standards were established for medical education and physician licensing, and alternative healers were suppressed. Physicians were hired as state health officers, gaining administrative and regulatory power. In Germany, many of the federated states adopted the same approach until a national system of state licensure and education was established in the mid-1800s. In Britain the process took longer, but by the mid-nineteenth century unlicensed practitioners could be sued for assault or manslaughter and the government could hire only registered physicians for state positions. American medical practice resisted organization until the 1870s, when a few states began to require a medical education for physician licensure. By the beginning of the twentieth century, American physicians were roughly on par with their European colleagues.

Throughout the nineteenth century, knowledge of the body's structure and processes had improved, tightening the relationship of medical practice to scientific findings and Koch's germ theory of disease. In the 1800s the human body came to be seen in a mechanical light, and human physiological processes were increasingly subject to deliberate experimental manipulation. Tools and scopes were introduced that Hays says "enabled their users to pose as detached observers of the body," measuring temperature, blood pressure, and pulse. Anesthetic gases revolutionized surgery between 1845 and 1855, and since "the patient no longer howled and writhed in agony, the surgeon could be meticulous." Acceptance of germ theory completed the process of objectifying disease, because germs came to be seen as separate organisms that caused disease by invading an otherwise-healthy body. Disease became an external enemy that could be conquered. Ironically, physicians benefited greatly from public acceptance of the germ theory and subsequent introduction of vaccinations, ideas they had loudly discounted until the late 1870s.

However, in rural areas, where physicians were remote or too expensive, alternative healers continued to hold sway. Resistance came from other quarters as well. The germ theory challenged patterns of etiological thought that Hays says had been undisturbed since the triumph of Christianity in the old Roman empire. When Pope Pius IX declared in an 1864 encyclical that he did not have to "reconcile himself with progress, liberalism, and modern civilization," he gave free rein to Catholic cults of miraculous healing. Due to slow formalization of licensure requirements, alternative healing systems flourished in the United States. Homeopathy gained popularity, and the Christian Science and Seventh Day Adventist churches enjoyed wide followings. Patent medicines were marketed by itinerant traders with slogans, pictures, trademarks, and their manufacturers positioned them as healthful and natural alternatives to physician-prescribed remedies with chemical and mineral components such as mercury. Many of today's large pharmaceutical companies had their start producing patent medicines, and Hays says that "physicians, even with modern scientific education, had trouble keeping up with the pharmacological sophistication of Friedrich Bayer's giant works" in Germany. Bayer's aspirin, introduced in 1899, was not only profitable but effective, a claim that could not be made for many patent formulas, including William Radam's Microbe Killer. The Texan's formula—concocted of water, wine, and hydrochloric and sulfuric acids—was introduced in the 1880s and was wildly successful.

Between 1870 and 1885, as more and more of the microbes underlying specific diseases were identified, the germ theory gained adherents. Pasteur's successful demonstration of his anthrax vaccine for cattle and sheep in 1881 won more converts, but vaccine demonstrations on human subjects were delayed until Pasteur successfully treated a boy bitten by a rabid dog with his newly developed rabies vaccine. Governments favored vaccines because they provided an alternative to difficult and expensive sanitation and housing projects for the poor, making social transformation and redistribution of economic resources unnecessary.

Before World War I, the transition to low mortality in the West had gone through three stages that had little to do with organized medicine. From 1730 to 1820 mortality fell when the plague disappeared, coinciding with a drop in global temperature known as the Little Ice Age. Nutrition improved as agricultural technology developed, cities were cleaner and had better drainage, and mothers practiced safer infant care and feeding. Deaths from smallpox declined because the disease became less virulent with widespread inoculation campaigns. Then the adverse health effects of rapid urbanization caused mortality gains to plateau from 1820 to the mid-nineteenth century. Overloaded sanitation systems contributed to increases in waterborne diseases such as diarrhea, dysentery, cholera, and typhoid, and urban crowding increased airborne infections such as tuberculosis, diphtheria, measles, and influenza. Even with these setbacks, death rates did not spike upward as they had in earlier periods, and after a temporary hiatus, mortality began another steep decline from 1870 to World War I, with falling tuberculosis rates, better housing, reliable piped water and modern sanitation.

After World War I and the subsequent influenza epidemic of 1918, human longevity began a steady rise in developed countries that continues to this day. Up until the late nineteenth century, women's life expectancy had been suppressed by poor nutrition and deaths in childbirth. Nationalistic pro-birth propaganda pushed young mothers to increase birth rates and improve child rearing practices in the years before World War I to counter dwindling supplies of soldiers in European states. Women benefited from improved living conditions, home sanitation standards, and hygiene during childbirth, and for the first time in human history, their life expectancy exceeded that of males. Diphtheria, scarlet fever, and whooping cough declined in virulence, and generations of exposure had increased immunity to tuberculosis.

By the end of the nineteenth century, the medical professional had achieved considerable status, even though scientific medicine developed too late to claim much credit for improved health or the decline of epidemics in the nineteenth century West.[4] Medical interventions were relatively futile until the late 1800s, and even the few effective interventions were not widely available until after World War I. Vaccines for anthrax, smallpox, typhoid, and rabies, developed in the late 1800s, did not become widely available until after the war, and vaccines for diphtheria, tetanus, and tuberculosis were not developed until the 1920s. Vaccines for typhus, whooping cough, yellow fever, and influenza were not available until World War II. The polio vaccine was developed in 1955, and vaccines for measles, mumps, and rubella were developed in the 1960s. Penicillin, discovered by Alexander Fleming in 1928, was not manufactured until 1943, because manufacturers were focusing on sulfonamide drugs. When its superior power to kill microbial parasites was recognized, penicillin quickly replaced sulfa drugs that could only arrest the microbial action. Discovery of sister antibiotics actinomycin and strepto-mycin followed in 1944, and discovery of isoniazid and the broad-spectrum antibiotics auremycin and chloramphenicol in the 1950s encouraged rapid development of more antibiotics by pharmaceutical giants interested in the enormous profits to be had from lifesaving drugs.

❋   ❋   ❋

By the early twentieth century, writes University of London expert Richard Evans, "the age of epidemics in western Europe was largely over." The work of European medical genius now lay in its colonies, where improvement of health and mitigation of suffering would be the "gift" of empire. The "con-quest" of disease in European states was the wonder of the world, and European medicine was ready to go to war on behalf of the "aboriginals." In 1926 Frenchman Hubert Lyautey proclaimed, *"La seule excuse de la colonisa-tion c'est la médecin,"* (the only excuse for colonization is the doctor). By the time colonial medicine was organized, however, European contact had had such a devastating effect on the native populations of the Pacific, the Americas, Australia, and Africa, it was impossible for medicine to scratch the surface of repair. The scale of deaths among the Ameridians in the sixteenth century was matched in the next two centuries by contact deaths on other continents, including Africa. Disease and the white man's arrival were associated so closely in the minds of Cook Islanders in the 1830s that they became "shippy" when they fell ill. As the intensity of European conquest increased from the late eighteenth to early twentieth centuries, the epidemiological, demographic, environmental, and social impact on colonial populations worsened. Roads, railroads, labor migration, military recruitment, and civilian enterprise broke coastal barriers, destroying the protection against imported diseases provided by distance and slow land transportation. The influenza epidemic of 1918 spread along these lines of contact in Africa with frightening speed.

Colonial military campaigns in Asia and Africa re-created the conditions of medieval Europe, when unwashed soldiers, auxiliaries, porters, and camp followers spread diseases, including a new one the Indians called *firangi roga*, the European disease, syphilis. Harsh European military and civilian labor recruitment campaigns caused higher mortality than earlier slaving expeditions. Mining and factory towns were as unsanitary and crowded as the cities of Industrial Age Europe, becoming centers for transmission of air- and waterborne infections and STDs, carried back to rural compounds by migrant workers. Besides introducing new diseases, European colonial incursions created devastating ecological changes in Africa. Mining, plantation agriculture, irrigation schemes, and drainage ditches created good habitats for malaria-bearing mosquitoes. As Africans died from smallpox and famine, cultivated areas returned to bush, promoting the spread of tsetse flies and, with them, sleeping sickness. Disease cleared the way in Africa and Asia for European colonization as it had in the sixteenth century Americas, crushing military resistance and emptying lands for white farming and settlement. Historian Alfred Crosby called this displacement "biological imperialism," whereby European crops, animals, and diseases displaced local flora, fauna, and people.

To the colonized, epidemics and accompanying disasters were manifestations of divine judgment and colonial malevolence unleashed against troublesome races. The concurrence of epidemic catastrophe with European conquest deepened the bewilderment and trauma of conquest. For their part, Europeans prided themselves on their scientific understanding of disease causation and mocked the fatalism, superstition, and barbarity of native responses to disease. The generalized ill health of colonial populations, especially in Africa, caused by severely debilitating chronic diseases like malaria, sleeping sickness, and bilharzia, contributed to the image of the native as lazy, less "fit" in the Darwinian sense, and inferior. European popular and medical opinion decided that illness was a sign of moral and social sickness in its subject populations.

For colonial administrations, medicine was an entry point, a way to get the information they needed to rule and modernize their subjects. Public health justified interference in the daily lives of native peoples, and the colonialists' demands to change traditional practices "for their own good." Campaigns against sleeping sickness, plague, cholera, yellow fever, and malaria became aggressive after 1890. The sudden proliferation of medical power was central to the development of colonial states and economies. Subject populations responded with no more enthusiasm to these invasions than the native poor had at home. Contrasting earlier epidemic responses in colonial Asia and Africa can help us understand why disease is so much more entrenched today in Africa than it is in Asia.

�

�"Xincompatible"

✻ ✻ ✻

The Asian subcontinent included some of the oldest, most populous, complex, and richest civilizations in the world, and Asian rulers retained control over their societies in the face of European intrusion. The possibility of eradicating native Asians and replacing them with European settlers, as had occurred in Africa and other regions of the world, was small. In the words of Jo Hays, "European migrants could never be more than foam on the surface of society." In Asia, European conquest was not facilitated by disease as it had been in the Americas, where there also had been complex and rich civilizations, because the disease burden of Europe and Asia had been shared over many thousands of years. Unlike Oceania and the Americas, this was not virgin soil for European diseases. In fact, Asia was often the source of the diseases most feared by Europeans. Unlike Africa, where native peoples were taken as slaves and soldiers and their lands converted to plantations, in Asia political and economic structures were never completely taken over, and social and economic changes proceeded much more gradually.

Asia had rich, well-informed, and effective systems of healing at the time of European contact. Although Britain initially approached Indian traditional healing with respect, the Sepoy Rebellion of 1857 brought about a radical change in British thinking about India and its culture. A British order to use a new type of grease on firearms provoked such a widespread rebellion among the largely vegetarian Hindu troops who thought they were being poisoned by animal fat that it almost cost the British their control. They became more careful about confronting native cultural beliefs, and the rebellion convinced them that "India was beyond redemption and that British rule could aim only at lofty trusteeship of the unregenerate barbarians," Hays says. It also made the British more determined to protect the basic health of their troops, and in the 1860s drainage, water supply, and sanitation were improved in barrack towns. The British also began to segregate themselves residentially from the native population.

In 1868 Britain and other European governments labeled India the homeland of cholera and urged the Indian government to curtail the movement of pilgrims within the country to reduce epidemic transmission. British development of railway lines and roads greatly facilitated the rapid spread of epidemics within the country, but the potential for rebellion made the government cautious about controlling pilgrims' movements. In the 1880s, when Turkey and France asked British India to prohibit pilgrims from traveling to Mecca to prevent the spread of cholera, British colonial and Indian business interests resisted interference and quarantine. Bombay medical authorities created the first medical laboratory in the country to refute Koch's claims concerning the bacteriological transmission of cholera. In the meantime, the health impact of major water, sewer, and drainage systems built in Calcutta were mixed, and municipal governments in many other parts of the country refused to increase taxation to finance similar infrastructure.

As new waves of cholera began having less effect on other areas of the world because of the Koch-inspired interventions, the British administration largely ignored new outbreaks of cholera and plague in India in the late 1800s and early 1900s. Hays says the apathy was "borne partly of racist complacency; the disease, though it ultimately killed 12 million Indians, was not spreading as a new Black Death to the West." Riots broke out against plague control measures. Devout Hindus resisted efforts to eliminate rat populations, compounding British anxieties about undertaking active disease control programs. The British were also confounded by the complexity of the disease environment, where malaria, tuberculosis, smallpox, and influenza also were killing huge numbers of Indians.

Frustrated by their inability to undertake major measures for disease control, the British attempted to involve local leaders more fully and to respect Hindu sensitivities, but without the money for a more comprehensive "public health police state," they were doomed to piecemeal efforts. Since a massive sanitation campaign was not possible, the British maintained even greater social distance from the natives, but the British in India would "never be safe so long as the native population and its towns and villages are left uncleansed to act as a reservoir of dirt and disease," the sanitary commissioner reported in 1894. The task of "cleansing" the subcontinent was too gigantic to contemplate. The British were unwilling to bear either the cost or the political risks because such a project required them "to meddle deeply

and dangerously in the habits and customs of the natives," says Indian
historian Ravi Chandavarkar.

✵ ✵ ✵

In the late 1800s, Africa's epidemic environment was typical of colonial
contact areas all over the world, but the alternation of disease and famine in
Africa perpetuated social conditions that had long been surpassed elsewhere.
Unlike Asia, Africa's major civilizations had already collided with slavers and
with one another, and colonization was the last, fatal blow. The late nineteenth and early twentieth centuries were "a peculiarly unhealthy time" in
east and central Africa, Ransford says, when millions died. There is no
absolute record of the population losses resulting from European contact, but
some idea of the effect can be gained from "before and after" data from two
colonial areas. The population of the Belgian Congo, estimated at 40 million
before 1880, dropped to 15.5 million by 1910 and to 9.25 million in 1933.
In one French West African colony, population dropped from 20 million in
1911 to 2.5 million in 1931.

The collision of diseases in Africa involved animals as well as people. Until
1890 the Serengeti Plain had been a relatively balanced ecosystem. Plants,
animals, people, and microorganisms coexisted successfully in a flourishing
and diverse ecology. The tsetse fly, harmless to wild ungulates and native cattle, prevented large-scale human presence, except for small groups of Masai
and Sukuma with their small herds of native cattle. The British, who arrived
in East Africa in 1884, and the Italians, who attempted to invade Ethiopia in
1889, brought cattle infected with rinderpest virus from the Black Sea area
of Asia. The virus was unknown in Africa, and within two years most of the
native domestic cattle and wild ungulates were dead. These animals had con-
stituted the primary food sources of the Masai, who were reduced to chew-
ing the bark of trees. Weakened by starvation, they were swept down by
smallpox. Lions, which had lost their natural prey, attacked the survivors,
who fled, abandoning their villages. While the populations of ungulates
revived, the rinderpest virus erupted once every ten years between 1917 and
1959, killing off entire populations of buffalo, wildebeest, giraffe, and Masai
cattle. Finally, a vaccination program in 1952 protected the native cattle, and
by the early 1960s, rinderpest disappeared. Sleeping sickness, however,
still hangs on in the acacia thickets that are an essential part of this delicately
balanced ecosystem.

Early colonial medical departments were obsessed with finding ways to prevent the spread of diseases, but their medical campaigns were underfunded

because colonial government budgets were usually small and provided health services only to the white minorities. As the British did in India, African colonial administrations made use of a number of techniques, including segregation of sleeping sickness victims and killing rats to fight bubonic plague. Many campaigns were launched between the 1890s and World War I against sleeping sickness, plague, cholera, yellow fever, and malaria— massive exercises in intervention and social manipulation that interfered directly in the lives of subject people.

The military often helped with the campaigns, contributing to the confusion of people who were forcibly removed from their home areas, neighbors, and families to prevent the spread of disease. The French, Americans, and Belgians organized mobile medical battalions that were unhindered by red tape or cultural sensitivity. The military's earlier extensive expeditions had punished resistors to the hut tax by systematically destroying crops and people, causing famines and triggering epidemics. Natives viewed the military's interest in public health as suspicious because the armed forces had suppressed uprisings across the continent with brutal force. As in Europe during the Black Death and nineteenth-century cholera epidemics, disease control measures included destruction or collection of property and animals, personal searches, and forcible confinement that often provoked riots. Although the devastating impact of the 1918 influenza epidemic heightened suspicions about the effectiveness of European medicine, military-style disease campaigns continued into the 1950s.

Tropical epidemics posed a constant threat to the economic and political viability of the early colonies, and repeated cholera epidemics made it clear that uncontrolled disease could threaten Europe itself. International pressure was brought to bear on colonial governments because high levels of epidemic mortality were a mark of poor colonial management. According to Hays, medicine was used "to deflect international criticism from the more sordid aspects of empire" and "provided a vehicle for thorough social and political control of a potentially fractious colony." Western medicine matured at just the right time to be used as a "tool of empire," allowing European penetration into areas that had been closed by disease barriers. In 1905 the United States undertook a massive campaign that lasted until 1913 to eradicate yellow fever in Central America so it could build the Panama Canal. In Africa, colonial medicine emphasized the health of workers in mines, barracks, factories, and cities, ignoring rural areas and favoring quick treatment rather than prevention. For the same reasons, North American capitalists invested in malaria and hookworm eradication to improve labor productivity in the American South.

The link between malaria and mosquitoes was not identified by Ronald Ross until 1898, after Alphone Laveran identified the malaria plasmodium in 1880 and the Scottish doctor Patrick Manson demonstrated the links between filariasis and mosquitoes in the late 1870s. Manson headed a civilian hospital serving expatriates in Amoy, China, along with the nearby missionary hospital that catered to the Chinese. Intrigued by the elephantitis he saw in many of his Chinese patients, while on leave in London he read reports from French West Africa of small snakelike worms (microfilaria) in the scrotal sac of an elephantitis patient. Manson returned with a microscope, and after determining that the number of microfilaria in his patients surged in the early evening when they were most likely to be bitten by mosquitoes, he realized the role of the mosquito in transmitting disease. Manson's research on elephantitis inspired subsequent research on malaria, and the Cuban physician Carlos Finlay y Barres identified the link between yellow fever and mosquitoes in the late 1870s, although the search for a bacterial cause delayed treatment until after 1900.

Before 1800 European traders had sought the services of local healers who were familiar with local diseases. The Spanish used local remedies in the Americas, most notable cinchona bark, and the Portuguese visited Hindu Ayurvedic practitioners in India. In 1622 the British East India Company advocated that local employees use Indian medicine rather than more expensive imported medicines, because "the Indies hath drugs in far greater plenty and perfection than here." During the late nineteenth century, however, European attitudes toward local medicine changed with advances in disease control in Europe. Both the Dutch and British East India companies employed European physicians and surgeons and established hospitals for European colonial settlements. In London and Liverpool, schools of tropical medicine were created in 1899, and courses were introduced in other medical schools on the continent and in the United States. Tropical doctors enjoyed growing prestige, linked with their wide authority to mandate colonial public health measures. Well-known specialists visited colonial administrations to advise them on medical matters, and boards of inquiry were assembled to address specific epidemics, such as the plague in India in 1899 and sleeping sickness in Uganda in 1902. Tropical doctors were linked through international congresses called to monitor the spread of infectious diseases among countries.

European medical science used Africa as a "diseased environment" ripe for research. Africa was a laboratory to test the new bacteriology, a place where scientific reputations could be made. One-fifth of all newly trained medical graduates left Britain for practices in tropical and subtropical climates after six months of training to investigate insect-borne and other exotic diseases. Most were more interested in biology and ecology than medicine. Worse, the importance of sanitation was marginalized, replaced by medical research campaigns and "the relentless pursuit of the pathogen," according to tropical disease expert Meredith Turshen. But in Africa, an essential piece was missing from the puzzle Koch and Pasteur had managed to put together in Europe. For some tropical diseases the pathological agent and routes of transmission could be easily identified, but for others the pathogen had not yet been identified and the causal chain was unknown.

In 1903 Patrick Manson consolidated the *ad hoc* disease control efforts of British colonies around the world into the Colonial Medical Service, and medical training for African auxiliary staff began a few years later. The training centers in Abidjan, Kampala, and Harare evolved into full-fledged medical schools and research centers. Medical surveys were undertaken to establish the geographic distribution of diseases. Despite these efforts, many administrative, economic, and public health measures worked at cross-purposes. Colonial prices were so low that people hoarded their crops, which attracted rats. Labor conscription and movement often contributed to the transmission of diseases. The early smallpox vaccine was painful, although after Africans saw the effect of injections for yaws, they began to love "Mr. Jackson" (the injection), and colonial authorities enlisted village headmen and chiefs to run vaccination campaigns.

Missionaries provided much of the direct care in rural Africa because colonial governments lacked the money to provide health services to natives outside of urban areas, mines, and plantations. Private employers also financed prevention and care services once they saw the advantages of a healthy workforce. The first mission hospital in Africa was established in 1518 by missionaries in Mozambique, and Francisans had opened hospitals in Angola by the end of the 1500s. The London Missionary Society's first doctor, David Livingstone, set sail for Africa in 1840. Being a missionary was dangerous work. The Wesley Missionary Society sent 225 men to West Africa between 1835 and 1907, 35 of whom died, and the Baptist Missionary Society lost half of its missionaries between 1878 and 1888. In most of Africa, mission hospitals still provide about half of all medical services today.

Without medicine, missionaries faced an impenetrable barrier. Bishop Smythies of the British Universities Mission to Central Africa testified in 1893 that "there are some mission fields in which only doctors seem to be able to gain any great influence." Distrust of Christianity as the religion of empire was so profound that only through alleviating pain and suffering could missionaries hope to gain a hearing from the populations they strove to convert. Missionaries with medical backgrounds were enthusiastically recruited, and funds were raised to build hospitals and dispensaries and to provide drugs. In most of tropical Africa, it was the only care available outside of commercial centers and company doctors on plantations.

Missionaries linked physical healing to spiritual healing and proselytization and were at odds with colonial authorities about healing approaches, especially for STDs. Christian medical societies were responding to what they viewed as the physical and moral decay of Africa. Just as cholera in India was not only a disease, but an outcome of despised religious practices— Hindu pilgrimages and rituals—outbreaks of syphilis in Africa were exaggerated by missionary prejudice against the perceived promiscuity of the natives. To the missionaries themselves and the bourgeois society they represented, "the diseases of Africa stood for larger spiritual ills, the sick bodies of Africans for the sickness of their souls," says tropical disease expert Megan Vaughn. Missionaries wanted to change African ideas of fertility and child rearing because the first two decades of colonial rule had increased mortality rates among children and infertility rates among women. The missionaries also found that African children were "uncontrollable," so they tried to change child-rearing practices to make children more "civilized."

Mission society fundraising relied on negative images of the continent, so for "church-going Britons of this period one of the most popular representations of Africa and of Africans came via the accounts in missionary journals of the woes of the 'sick continent,' and the trials, tribulations, and triumphs of heroic medical missionaries," Vaughn says. Healing was part of a program of social and moral engineering to save Africans, and missionary reports fostered public perception of Africans as "sick," living on "sick continent," and people to be pitied and despised. This image dates back to David Livingstone, who, when he "opened up" central Africa, found it "wounded" by the slave trade and wanted to heal it, and still colors our view of Africa. Missionaries did champion the cause of Africans threatened by European development policies and systems because they were worried that eastern and southern Africa's rural communities would die out between World Wars I and II. They criticized the harsh migrant labor system and extractive policies of colonial governments that had, during World War I, stripped Africa of too many resources. When the depression hit in the 1930s, colonial health expenditures were severely cut, and contributions to missionary societies also declined.

Experience in Africa showed there were no simple solutions to the multiple disease problems of African populations because poverty and malnutrition were intractably linked to disease outbreaks on the continent. In 1933 the League of Nations' *Report on Nutrition and Public Health* in member countries found that colonial populations were undernourished due to their backwardness and ignorance. The official report was a whitewash of the real findings of colonial medical officers who reported malnutrition levels so serious that treatment of disease, no matter how effective and widely carried out, would achieve negligible results. The British Colonial Department, under investigation in 1925 for nutritional problems associated with heavy colonial livestock losses, initiated another major survey of colonial malnutrition in 1936. It looked at the balance of subsistence and commercial farming promoted in its agricultural policies. Reports from the Caribbean, West Africa, and the Far East found that most cases of malnutrition among children occurred because their parents were unable to afford food due to the impact of the export-oriented colonial economies. The draft summary identified poverty as the main cause of malnutrition, "produced by inadequate production of food crops, low wages, and poor yields, and by colonies receiving insufficient returns for their export crops," all effects of extractive policies that had long been criticized by agricultural experts for their economic and ecological consequences.

When the home government realized that the report's recommendations would reduce produce imports from the colonies and raise their prices, the report was completely rewritten to eliminate any criticism of the colonial extraction policies and the economic and structural problems they created. The potentially incendiary conclusions of the draft report were buried, and the final report stressed native ignorance and general backwardness. Malnutrition was officially viewed as an endemic problem for which colonialism had little responsibility and over which it could exercise little control.

Responsibility for all of Africa's disease problems were systematically deflected away from colonial powers onto the "backwardness" and "cultural practices" of the natives themselves, and medicine helped create Africa "as a repository of death, disease, and degeneration," says Vaughn. Since most medical interventions had failed, social and cultural explanations for disease patterns were sought and formed the basis of wider "knowledge of 'the African,'" a dynamic that still features strongly in constructing strategies to deal with HIV/AIDS. Africans were portrayed as beyond understanding and beyond help, a message colored by the fact that it was carried to Europe and the United States by missionaries, who exaggerated the situation to raise money for their work. They saw themselves as men and women "grappling with a wild and uncontrolled environment, of which Africans were an integral part," Vaughn says. Colonial psychologists even "denied the possibility that Africans might be self-aware individual subjects, so bound were they by collective identities."

Despite the propaganda, most colonial medical officers fully understood the underlying causes of epidemics. The director of medical services in southern Nyasaland (modern Malawi) argued that an epidemic of cerebrospinal meningitis among laborers in the 1930s could be addressed only through improved living conditions. Most were convinced that substandard living conditions and structural deficiencies of employment contributed to regular epidemics, but still sought to change cultural practices to protect health. W. T. C. Berry, the medical officer of southern Malawi's Mulanje district, argued that changes in funerary practices and maintenance of sexual taboos were essential to reduce outbreaks of meningitis. When a young man asked if he could sleep with his wife after Berry's lecture on meningitis, the doctor advised abstinence for several weeks to avoid infection.

The inability of colonial medicine to repair the ravages of colonization in Africa, its subsequent cynicism, manipulation of African reality, and readiness to blame the victim was part of a vast exercise in Social Darwinism that harmed people like Molly, Pauline, and Robina and their communities as much as it helped them. The same drama is being played out now with the HIV/AIDS epidemic in sub-Saharan, but political and economic motivations have been brought to a conscious level. The epidemic has made us more sensitive to the plight of have-nots and more aware of the impact of our role in their deprivation and its impact on their survival.

But our willingness to help still depends on whether we feel threatened. History shows that the more distant a disease threat seems and the less likely it is to infect us, the less likely we are to respond. Deliberately encouraging the deaths of the world's poor, or a lack of compassion for them, as was the case with New World Native Americans, Oceanic islanders, or Australian aborigines at the time of colonial contact is no longer acceptable. But the alternative of sitting passively by in the face of massive death and destruction of people on a different continent is still possible in the modern world, as our inaction on HIV/AIDS demonstrates. As we shall see in the next chapter, human responses to epidemics of STDs are even more convoluted because of their highly charged relationship to reproduction and sex.

CHAPTER SIX

Sexually Transmitted Diseases

The chiefs were drifting in and taking their places. Molly looked at her watch. It was exactly nine-thirty. Robina welcomed them, and some of the chiefs agreed to talk about the problems families were facing in their villages. "Don't go on too long," Robina advised them. "Highlight the most important problems." She looked at her watch, embarrassed. "I wonder what's keeping our friends from the NACP and Save the Children? It's almost ten o'clock." One of the senior chiefs grunted. "I guess we know who's important around here." "Maybe they had some car trouble," Robina said cheerfully. "They're coming from Kampala, and last week the road was still being repaired."

The car screeched up just as she was finishing. The National AIDS Control Program staff scurried in and began distributing flyers and condoms. Molly looked at Pauline. "Don't tell me they're going to do a condom demonstration here," she croaked. "We've got the church choir coming in to start the meeting, and some of those children are very young." "Never too early to start," Pauline said, looking grim. "I mean, teaching them what they need to know. We're going to have to live with this thing for a long time, and most of them have been playing sex in the bush since they hit puberty."

When Robina introduced Dr. Okware, the National AIDS Control Program director, he looked Pauline up and down closely. "I think he wants a blanket," she whispered to Molly behind her hand, and they both started to giggle. "These Ganda men are randy boys." "What do you expect when they start teaching us how to please men before we even know what a penis is really for?" Molly laughed. "When my mother started to tell me . . . ." She broke off as Robina cleared her throat. The AIDS Control staff finished setting up the projector and were running the electric cord to the generator. Robina leaned toward Dr. Okware. "Could we start your part now and let Save the Children catch up when they get here?" After his assistants readied the overhead projector, he began to drone.

"AIDS," he said, "is a new disease in Uganda. Toward the end of 1982 several local traders—you might know them," he joked, "who engaged in illicit trade and smuggling across the border died at Kasensero fishing village on Lake Victoria. This was almost two years after the disease had been reported in the United States and elsewhere in Africa. When they died the population took it lightly, because it was believed that such misfortune was a result of natural justice against cheats and smugglers. Decent businessmen smiled, but the smiles stopped when spouses of AIDS victims started dying. Everyone got concerned; the survivors fled inland to towns, taking with them the infection. Many spent sleepless nights, especially those who had affairs with prostitutes."[1]

Several of the chiefs were inspecting the hands folded in their laps rather closely. Molly noted with pleasure that the chief from Kabula seemed to be awake and was not playing with his pencil. Abdul Rashid was attentive; the young man from Byakabanda was one of Robina's favorites and had started organizing orphan committees in the villages of his area before it had been formally proposed to the chiefs' council.

The choir had finished its second round of songs, and several fourteen-year-old girls sat wide-eyed as the AIDS Control education director slid a condom on a penis model. The chiefs were fumbling with their own practice versions, and everyone was grimly serious. "I'm glad the young girls are learning now," Pauline commented quietly to Molly. "I learned the hard way when I was their age from one of my uncles. I hurt for days after my first sex play, and I avoided him so carefully my mother asked what was wrong. I just burst into tears. She gave him a stern lecture and sent him down the road. He'd been 'visiting' from Masaka."

"I think Save the Children is finally here!" Molly whispered, putting her hand on Pauline's arm. "And just in time! I thought Wallace was going to launch into his own lecture any minute." Robina called for the tea break, and everyone headed for the door. "Oh, no!" Pauline said. "Here comes Dr. Williams from the Columbia Research Project. He's asked me so many questions about dry sex, I think he's going to start a club when he goes back to New York City. Think I'll go get some tea." Molly nodded. "Think I'll go with you. What I know about traditional Baganda sex practices can be fit inside a cup."

Save the Children's tall dark-haired social welfare officer started his speech after the break by apologizing to the group. "We were held up by the road construction work in the swamps just southwest of Kampala," he explained, and introduced his two Ugandan assistants, social welfare graduates from Makerere. "I'm sure you all know them both, and you probably also know Susan Hunter." The small, dark-haired woman rose and smiled, nodding at the chiefs she had visited during the orphan enumeration. "Susan has started writing up some of the findings from your work but is anxious to get the rest of your reports, so she and Charles and James can computerize them." Mrs. Nyeko smiled at Molly. It looked like things were headed in the right direction.

When Robina finished presenting the orphan reports, Chief Rashid cleared his throat. "Mrs. Nyeko here," he nodded at Robina, "asked some of us to tell you what's going on in the villages." The response to AIDS in his county had been negative at first, but when he called the village chiefs together and told them about the disease, they started to help. "Now that people understand," he continued, "they're able to put things right. Peasants are always a pretty practical sort—I know, because when I can get the time away from Mrs. Nyeko's meetings and local funerals, I am one myself—and they are willing to accept the sufferers and their children now that they know they won't be infected. The villagers in my area are raising a communal garden and have asked for money to repair the school so they can eliminate fees for orphans."

He paused to clear his throat. "We've only had one serious incident," he continued, looking around him. "Most of you already heard about it. It's what convinced me I had to educate my constituents. One night a few people in Lwamwaga who believed that HIV was caused by witchcraft decided they would clean out the witches. They rounded up six—all women—and hung them all." He paused and looked straight at the Save the Children party. "It's a tragedy that I never want to see happen again, and I'm hoping you can help us avoid it. Molly's plan for OCBO—the Orphan Community Based Organization—is a solid one, and we want you to sponsor it in the entire district."

Robina blinked, taken aback by the grim way the proposal had been introduced. Well, she thought, at least it got their attention. "Yes," she said, "each of the chiefs has worked up a budget at the subcounty level, and the entire proposal can be funded for less than the cost of a Land Rover." Way less, she thought. "The total is $12,000 for the year, or about 30 cents a child." "You can carve a lot of penis models for that," Pauline whispered to Molly. "Of course, it's expensive because it includes prevention programs and penis models, but we're hoping Dr. Okware can send us the condoms we need." Molly thought the doctor winced, but Robina went on.

"Gentlemen—and ladies—this is another kind of war. We must have the resources, or our futures will be lost, and those of our children." Molly held her breath. What would they say?

✄ ✄ ✄

What Darwin had to say about sex in *The Origin of the Species* was, not surprisingly, very limited given Victorian squeamishness about the subject. The several-hundred-page-long work only devotes two pages to sexual selection, part of Darwin's discussion of natural selection, and only includes examples from other species: birds, fish, stags, and alligators. The main theme of his book was still so controversial that he probably decided to minimize any other topics that would raise Victorian hackles. By 1859, when *The Origin* was published, Darwin was fifty years old and had fathered seven children. While not a novice, his sexual experiences probably had been confined to his wife following their marriage, given their devotion, his busy work schedule, and his avoidance of city life. His elder brother, Erasmus, who lived in London, had abandoned his medical practice early on to assume the life of a well-heeled bachelor. He introduced Charles to London's literary and scientific circles, but after debating the matter in his personal journal, Darwin decided on the quiet joys of married life and settled down with his cousin Emma. His decision seems to have included lifelong faithfulness to her. Taking his water cures at Malvern, Darwin enjoyed his dinner conversations with female "patients" of the spa, but while others apparently used the setting for illicit liaisons, in his free time he penned letters to Emma and worked on his real passion, natural selection.

Sexual selection, Darwin tells us in *The Origin*, depends not on bloody group competition for food sources or territory, "but on a struggle between the individuals of one sex, generally the males, for possession of the other sex. The result is not death to the unsuccessful competitor, but few or no offspring." It ensures that the "most vigorous males, those which are best fitted for their places in nature, will leave the most progeny." Tests of strength are one way to ensure selection of "good" genes, and polygamous animals, where the male is in charge of a herd, have the worst of it. "Male alligators have been described as fighting, bellowing, and whirling around, like Indians at a war dance, for the possession of the female." Salmon duel, Darwin wrote, and "male stag-beetles sometimes bear wounds from the huge mandibles of other males" while the female "sits by, an apparently unconcerned beholder of the struggle, and then retires with the conqueror."

Even where victory is secured by other "special weapons" than brute strength, the successful male's genes are selected for future generations by his breeding success. Birds compete for females through the beauty of their singing and other peaceful displays, Darwin continued. "The rock-thrush of Giana, birds of paradise, and some others, congregate; and successive males display with the most elaborate care... their gorgeous plumage; they likewise perform strange antics before the females, which, standing by as spectators, at last choose the most attractive partner." Other special defenses were protective as well as attractive, like a male lion's mane, which cushioned his neck against attacks by competing males. Wallace thought Darwin was dead wrong about male displays, arguing that females are dull because they sat on nests and needed camouflage. He preferred "survival of the fittest," the battles and fights to the finish, a term Darwin did not like at all but eventually adapted in *The Origin*.

The mechanisms of sex and reproduction had to be left to scientists with different talents from Darwin's, although his theorizing renewed interest in explaining the inner workings of human inheritance through microscopic study. Microscopes had been in use from the seventeenth century, and in 1665 Robert Hooke called the pores he identified in slices of cork "cells." Improvements in the lens system of the instrument in the 1800s allowed one of Darwin's closest friends, Robert Brown, to identify the nucleus of a cell from the epidermis of an orchid and to determine that it was an essential part of cell growth. In 1838, Matthias Jakob Schleiden found that plant growth was due to an organism's ability to produce new cells. In 1869, three years after the Austrian monk Gregor Mendel presented his findings on plant crosses to the Brunn Natural Science Society, a Swiss chemist, Johann Friedrich Meischer, discovered a mysterious, acidic, phosphorous-rich compound in white blood cells that he called "nuclein" and that he thought might be the seat of heredity. When isolated and purified by chemists in 1889 it was identified as deoxyribose nucleic acid, or DNA, but it would not be recognized as the stuff of human genes for another sixty years.[2] While studying sea urchins in 1875, Oskar Hertwig observed the fusion of sperm and egg during fertilization. In 1888 Wilhelm Van Waldeyer identified the "hereditary particles," or threads in cells he was examining, as chromosomes, and with improved straining techniques, Theodore Boveri determined that they were living bodies, proved that each cell needed a full set of threads to develop, and in 1903 discovered that gametes each have the same number of chromosomes but the number contributed by the mother and the father were different.

By the time Darwin died in 1882, seventy-three years and four days after his birth, the gonococcus responsible for gonorrhea had been identified by a German dermatologist, Albert Neisser. In 1837 syphilis had been distinguished from gonorrhea by French venereologist Phillipe Ricord, who also identified the primary, secondary, and tertiary stages of syphilis. Rudolph Virchow, one of the leading figures in the development of modern germ theory, established that an infection with syphilis could be transferred by the blood to internal organs, and in 1876 cardiovascular syphilis was identified. By the early twentieth century it was known that syphilis could spread to the spinal cord, causing loss of coordination and paralysis, and to the brain, causing dementia. A physician of the day estimated that one-third to one-half of the mental institutions in the U.S. would be empty if a treatment could be found, but it was not found for another fifty years.

The Victorian era was a time of enormous social and technological change that included advances in the natural sciences, public health, microbiology, and world conquest. It was also a time of enormous change in social attitudes toward sexuality, a conservative swing from the more relaxed attitudes of the Regency period, when sexual and personal expression was unfettered. But change in attitudes was by no means universal, and our notion of the Victorian era as overwhelmingly prudish has been shaped by selective editing. Many of the manuals, books, playing cards, devices for sexual titillation, and advertisements for sexual pleasures that might have demonstrated the extent of Victorian appetites have long been purged by official repositories and anxious homeowners who did not want the neighbors to know what Uncle Harry did on his evening excursions.[3] Victorians produced "bisexual pornography in which the two heroes indulge in guiltless sex with each other before climbing into bed with the two heroines; the children's adventure starring a cross-dressing teenage boy; the advertisements that wooed people like you and me into meetings with personalities like Julia Pastrana the Baboon Lady, Miss Atkinson the Pig Woman, and the Bipenis Boy," says historian Matthew Sweet. Although Victorians purportedly dressed their piano legs in knickers so they would be less lascivious, in London's swank Burlington Shopping Arcade, "sex and shopping were pursued with equal enthusiasm—and transvestite boys were its specialty."

During England's early Victorian era, religious and social moralizing aimed at repressing sexuality through a drive for self-mastery and through social control over excess and "irregular" pre- and extramarital sex, culminating in a concern about prostitution that reached panic levels in the 1850s and early 1860s. With the passage of the Contagious Disease Act in 1866, prostitutes were detained for medical examination to protect soldiers and sailors (and ordinary men) from debilitation, but the 1860s witnessed a resurgence of sexual freedom for men, encouraged in the next two decades by the idea that men had natural sexual urges and drives that had to be satisfied, a sentiment that arose, in part, from the demonstration of human links to other species.

The curtain came down on this freedom for men in the early 1880s, when the Social Purity campaign decried the double standard and demanded male continence outside of marriage. Although the Contagious Disease Act was modified to reduce penalties for prostitution, men were expected to control themselves, an idea that was turned into a political slogan, "Votes for Women, Chastity for Men" by Christabel Pankhurst, one of Britain's early suffragettes. Syphilis had been an important disease in Europe since the 1500s, but it was not until sexual permissiveness brought the disease home— "the virginal bride (and her innocent offspring) infected with syphilis by a sexually experienced husband"—that gender inequities were seen as threatening family life in England. Similar movements were afoot on the European continent and in the United States, but there were still cross-currents and many who argued that sex was a natural force beneficial to humans who pursued it. Far from being of one mind about repression of sexuality, the Victorian era was, until the late 1890s, a battlefield of opposing views about appropriate sexual expression. But Pankhurst won the day in 1885 with a bill that not only repealed the registration of prostitutes but made pornography and homosexuality illegal.

❊ ❊ ❊

Sexually transmitted diseases (STDs) have had profound—although unrecognized—effects on all societies since the introduction of syphilis to Europe by Columbus' sailors in 1492. They quickly spread world wide after being brought to Europe—a testament to the pervasive drive for sex that is part of humankind's basic survival instinct—and thrived, like other diseases, in the profound chaos of late medieval Europe and contemporary societies on other continents. Their impact as causes of widespread illness, disability, and death has been profound long before HIV/AIDS emerged in the 1980s. In addition to HIV, seven major sexually transmitted or venereal diseases (STDs, VDs, also called sexually transmitted infections, or STIs) have been identified since Ricord separated the first two, syphilis and gonorrhea, in 1837. Three are ulcerous: chancroid, genital herpes, and syphilis; and four are nonulcerous: chlamydia, papillomavirus, trichomoniasis, and gonorrhea. In addition to these seven major types, there are many other milder types of STDs resulting from bacterial or yeast infection, such as vaginitis and urethritis, and several skin conditions transmitted by lice, such as scabies. The first seven are the most dangerous, however, because they spread through the body to cause serious, even life-threatening problems. Syphilis caused 197,000 deaths in the world in 2001, chlamydia caused 7,000, and gonorrhea caused 4,000; 101,000 of these deaths were in Africa, and 96,000 in Southeast Asia.[4]

Three of the major STDs (gonorrhea, syphilis, and chlamydia) are caused by bacteria, and most of the rest are caused by viruses. *Chlamydia trachomatis* is a parasitic bacterium that resembles a virus because it can not reproduce outside a living cell although it can be treated by antibiotics. Trichomoniasis is caused by a protozoa, a one-celled animal belonging to the lowest division of the animal kingdom. All STDs can be systemic; that is, like syphilis, they infect other body organs and processes, cause pelvic inflammatory disease in women, and can be passed to newborn children in the birthing process. At least one, papillomavirus, which causes genital warts, is now known to cause cervical and prostate cancer, and others may be associated with cancer as well. Chlamydia can lead to arthritis, and in May 2000 careful lab tests revealed a possible connection between chlamydia and arteriosclerosis and Alzheimer's disease. Finally, many STDs lead to sterility and others produce painful lesions that reduce the frequency of coitus. The tubal scarring of gonorrhea and chlamydia caused a high incidence of female infertility in the 1970s in the United States. Polycystic ovary disease, found in 3 to 12 percent of women in the United States, also is believed to be caused by a sexually transmitted infectious pathogen. All STDs increase the risk of HIV. Open ulcers ease its spread through contact, and both ulcerous and nonulcerous types increase the viral "shedding" of HIV in sperm and vaginal fluids up to ten times, resulting in a radically higher risk of transmission for each sexual contact. Also, in women, STDs attract T cells to the cervix, disrupting the mucosal barriers and easing HIV transmission.

During the 1990s, the United States reduced gonorrhea and syphilis to their lowest-ever recorded rates, but Americans still have the highest rate of STDs of any developed country in the world, largely due to high rates of sexual activity. To take one example, the rate of gonorrhea, the second most prevalent STD in the United States, is twenty-six times higher than in Germany. Prevalence in the developing world is higher, but the statistics are not as good. STDs are rampant in young people because their elevated sex drives lead to higher rates of sexual activity, higher rates of partner change, and lack of knowledge and failure to use protection. In 1996 the incidence of chlamydia in U.S. females fifteen to twenty-four years of age was as high as 10.9 percent in some states, official rates experts know are significantly below the actual numbers. One in five adult Americans of any age carries the herpes simplex virus, which has increased 30 percent overall since 1970, but 500 percent among white teenagers. Half of all fifteen to forty-nine-year-old women in the United States are infected with the papilloma virus, including 34 percent of college-age women.

STD levels in the United States and other countries are high because many infections go undetected and unreported. They are symptomless, especially in women, have chronic but bearable symptoms, or cause the sufferer too much embarrassment to seek care. STDs have been called the "hidden epidemic" of the United States because most healthcare providers do not routinely screen their patients, especially males. In 2001 state health departments in the United States reported 783,000 cases of chlamydia, 362,000 cases of gonorrhea, and 6,000 cases of syphilis, but actual rates were much higher. Infections that are detected will not lead to death or advanced symptoms if treatment is available, but undetected infections can cause a host of severe biological and mental problems. Minority populations are especially vulnerable. While primary and secondary syphilis declined drastically in blacks and Hispanics during the 1990s, they still have three times the number of cases as whites.

※ ※ ※

The antiquity of venereal disease is not as easy to establish as the antiquity of other diseases because syphilis is the only STD that leaves telltale marks on bones. "After examining something like 30,000 bodies of ancient Egyptians and Nubians representing every period of the history of the last sixty centuries and from every part of that country," says paleontologist Elliott Smith, "it can be stated quite confidently that no trace whatever, even suggesting syphilitic injuries to bones or teeth, was revealed in Egypt before modern times." Marks found on Iron Age remains from southern Africa proved to be yaws, which has the same bacterial causal agent, *Treponema pallidum.* Syphilis is the only one of four related bacterial diseases called treponematoses that has achieved global distribution, possibly because of its felicitous mode of transportation. It is caused by Treponema S. The others—yaws (Treponema Y), pinta (Treponema C), and bejel (Treponema M)—are skin diseases with widespread distribution in different parts of the tropics. All Treponema varieties look the same under a microscope and reveal their differences only when they cause different diseases in their human hosts, depending in part on whether the setting is temperate or tropical.

Fallopius, the Italian anatomist and contemporary of Columbus, wrote that "amongst the Genoese was Christopher Columbus, a Man of remarkable Genius [sent] by Ferdinand and Isabella to the West Indies [where he found] most precious Gold, and great Plenty of it was brought from thence, together with an Abundance of Pearls." But, Fallopius continued, "there was also a thorn joined to the Rose, and Aloes mixed with the Honey. For Columbus brought back his Vessels laden with the French Disease. There the disease is like a mild Itch amongst us, but transplanted hither it is become so fierce and unmerciful, as to infect and corrupt the Head, Eyes, Nose, Palate, Skin, Flesh, Bones, Ligaments and at last the whole Bowels."

When they were bored, Columbus's sailors amused themselves by raping Hispaniola's Taino women, who had contracted yaws at an early age from their playmates. "While each rape was in progress, the long-unwashed and probably tender skin on Spanish groins, bellies, chests, and penises was breached by *Treponema pertenue*, the yaws causal agent," which mutated to *Treponema pallidum* when it reached cooler temperatures in Europe, says historian Sheldon Watts. Europe may have had a milder form of yaws— Roman bones were marked by lesions of the disease—and Columbus brought the new, more virulent strain back. Or the strain brought back by Columbus mutated and evolved independently in Europe. Two strains of a disease often coexist in a population—even in the same body—and the more virulent strain takes over when conditions are ripe.

Racism's expression in brutal imperial subjugation was perfected in the New World by Columbus, according to his first biographer, Bartolomé de las Casas, whose father sailed with Columbus on his second trip to the New World. After growing up on the Hispaniola plantation established by his father and becoming a slaveholder himself, Bartolomé became passionately antislavery and spent the remainder of his life defending Native Americans. Columbus recommended to Ferdinand and Isabella that the beautiful and gentle natives he met be kept captive on their own islands; "with fifty men you will keep them all in subjugation and make them do anything you wish," he said of one island's inhabitants. Despite his seeming appreciation for the Taino, he chopped an ear off one of his Indian prisoners on his second return voyage, an action that Las Casas said "was the first case of injustice perpetrated here in the Indies on the mistaken and vain assumption that what was being enacted was justice. It marked the beginning of the spilling of blood, later to become a river of blood, first on this island and then in every corner of these Indies."

When Columbus returned to Hispaniola in the fall of 1494, he retaliated against native rebellions by massacring the most recalcitrant Indians and shipping another 500 Taino back to Seville to be sold as slaves. He then marched across the island, razing villages and murdering inhabitants with guns, swords, and dogs trained to rip natives apart, a torture Las Casas described as "thought up, invented, and put into effect by the Devil."

Columbus also required that each adult pay a set measure of gold dust every three months, the beginnings of the hut tax. Columbus's "civilizing" and "development" measures claimed the lives of more than a third of Hispaniola's native population in two years, and in less than two generations, the remaining Taino had died from Spanish diseases. When some of his sailors rebelled during the third voyage, Columbus granted them each a piece of cultivable land and the natives living on it, but a judge sent by Ferdinand and Isabella to the island in 1500 was met by the sight of seven hanging Spaniards, executed for rebellion. Francisco de Bobadilla, the royal judge, immediately seized Columbus and shipped him back to Cadiz in chains. After some years spent wasting away with tuberculosis and following the Spanish court around demanding gratitude and recognition, Columbus died, bedridden and bitter. To Las Casas, it was divine justice, the just reward for a gratuitously cruel and ruthless man. And syphilis was indeed divine justice on the European imperialists, or at least tit for tat.

A New World origin of syphilis was first theorized in 1526, and by 1748, Enlightenment giant Charles de Secondat, Baron de Montesquieu took it for granted, associating the disease with European greed. "It was thirst for gold," he said, "which perpetuated this disease; people were continually going to America, each time bringing back new seeds." Whatever its origin, syphilis, which historian William McNeill suggests is a "historical analogue" for AIDS, has rivaled tuberculosis, cholera, smallpox, and the plague in the impact it has had on world civilization over the past five centuries. And like AIDS, it was responsible for a larger proportion of the death rate than ever actually recorded. Many of its victims succumb to heart disease or other medical problems. "Is it justifiable," a U.S. scientist asked in 1947, "to assume that syphilis actually ranks first, instead of its apparent tenth, among killing infections?"

❅ ❅ ❅

The world's first recorded outbreak of syphilis was in Naples, Italy, in 1493. The Spanish physician, Roderic Diaz, had treated several of Columbus' syphilitic sailors, including his pilot, Pinzon of Palos, and went on to write a thesis about it entitled *Fruit of All Saints Against the Disease of the Island of Espanola*. Diaz had first detected the "bubos," as the disease was then called because it produced pustules on the skin, in Barcelona in 1493. In fifteenth- and sixteenth-century Europe, where prostitutes were "pampered inmates of municipal brothels, part of the civic resources of the town" and serviced "captured" bridegrooms on the eve of their wedding, it did not take long before syphilis reached Naples through a coastal network of sailors and prostitutes. The city was under siege by 50,000 mercenaries from all corners of Europe in the hire of Valois France's Charles VIII, who claimed title to the city's throne. The mercenaries had "dallied for some weeks in papal Rome, where it was said that prostitutes outnumbered clerics," and invaded Naples with hardly any resistance because an epidemic of typhus was raging there. They cele- brated for several weeks, then withdrew to Fornovo near Milan, where they were disbanded, carrying syphilis with them and dispersing it throughout Europe.

Syphilis appeared in Germany by the summer of 1495, condemned by Holy Roman emperor Maximilian as an "evil pocks" that he blamed on the sin of blasphemy. It reached Switzerland and France in the same year, Holland, England, and Greenland a year later, and was reported in Hungary and Russia in 1499. By 1509 large numbers of Europeans from London to Moscow were "vexed with the frensshe pockes, poore, and nedy, leyenge by the hye wayes stykinge and almoost roten above the ground, suffering intollerably withe pus- cules & doloros burnings o the armis shulders nek & leggs or the shynnes as the bones shuld part from the flesh," according to a contemporary sermon.

The epidemic crossed to northern Africa with Jews and Muslims driven from Spain by Ferdinand and Isabella, where a contemporary observed that "if any Barbarie be infected with the disease commonly called the Frenche pox, they die thereof for the most part, and are seldom cured." It arrived in the Middle East by 1498. The Portuguese, among the earliest Europeans to get the pox, carried it the farthest, around the Cape of Good Hope to India under Vasco da Gama in 1498. It spread to Ceylon and the Malaysian penin- sula, and, traveling another coastal route, reached Canton in 1504—only a decade after it had left the Caribbean—where it was called the plum tree ulcer, and finally reached Japan in 1569. Since the fifteenth century, this "gift of the down-trodden natives of Espanola" has been the constant companion of civilized man.

When the new strain of syphilis began to spread in Europe, it was widely called the French pox, a reference to the soldiers who hastened its spread. Later the French called it the Italian pox, the Russians called it the Polish pox, and the Poles called it the German pox. Syphilis was named in 1530 by an Italian authority on the disease, who wrote a poem about a shepherd named Syphilis who committed so many acts of blasphemy that he caught the new pox, but the name did not become common until the eighteenth century. Before it was recognized as a venereal disease, the prevention measures advo- cated by Holy Roman emperor Maximilian I included prohibition of gambling, cursing, blasphemy, and other vices. When priests started coming down with it, breathing the air of an infected person was added to the list of causes. In his trial for treason, one of the most damning charges made against England's Thomas Cardinal Wolsey—who was infected with the French pox—was that he had breathed in the face of Henry VIII.

The sexual origin of the disease was recognized fairly quickly. Erasmus of Rotterdam described the mechanism of transmission in his *Colloquia* of 1523, and in his essay "A Marriage in Name Only," published six years later, he reported that spouses infected their mates, causing "both of them to rot alive, become paralysed or mad, and their offspring be born diseased or dead." By 1539, according to Ruy Diaz de Isla, a Lisbon surgeon, syphilis "has caused so much damage, that there is not a village in Europe with one hundred neighbors without ten of them dead of that ailment." An English doctor, William Clowes, estimated that in 1580 half of all the patients at the House of St. Bartholomew in London were syphilitic. Since most people shunned hospitals or could not afford them, hospital patients were probably only a small proportion of the total cases. While London may have been racked with syphilis, 80 percent of Britain's population then resided in the countryside, where "bastardy" rates were extremely low and sexuality was less pervasive.

As an entirely new disease in Europe, "its spectacular skin manifestations were massively contagious and quickly lethal." Historian Sheldon Watts speculates that at first, the epidemic was "a multiple-disease syndrome combining yaws, venereal syphilis, and gonorrhea." Over time, the thickening of the skin, bleeding, sores, and bone fractures of yaws dropped away, and as syphilis adapted to its new home, it became much less lethal. By 1519 syphilis sufferer Ulrich von Hutten wrote that "when it first appeared it caused a far more loathsome stench than it does now, as if the sickness involved were of a different type altogether." In the New World, where Native Americans were suffering from their first encounters with European measles, mumps, and chicken pox, a similar process of adaptation was occurring. These diseases were rarely life threatening in Europe, but Native Americans experienced tragic results, including paralysis, shingles, encephalitis, and orchitis (inflammation of the testes). Their children were born with severe birth defects, although they had been a much taller and healthier population than the European invaders at the time of contact.

Syphilis went through several waves of decreasingly severe symptoms, so by de Isla's time, the disease's bulbous pustules had been replaced by "gummy tumors." In its first stage of adaptation, 1494 to 1516, sufferers came down with a relatively mild body-rash that worsened quickly to destroy the palate, uvula, tonsils, and jaw, and created agonizing muscle and nerve pains. In the second period, lasting until 1526, syphilis added two new symptoms, severely painful bone inflammation with deterioration of the marrow and bone itself and genital warts or corns. In 1526, symptoms were reduced to pustules and swollen lymph glands in the groin, and after 1540, when the most spectacular symptoms began to die away, gonorrhea became a frequent companion of first-stage syphilis.

Hair and tooth loss was common among syphilitics, but it may have been a side effect of the only treatment known in the day, internal and external administration of mercury. Mercury's terrible side effects prompted von Hutten to remark that patients would be better off dying from the disease than taking the cure. Mercury poisoning may have contributed to the madness associated with syphilis, leading to widespread fear of witchcraft. It was reinforced by the rash of congenital diseases, malformations, and stillbirths caused by syphilis. Although cure was impossible in the absence of antibiotics, physicians' attempts to treat the disease made them rich. Physician Thierry de Héry, while kneeling before a statue of Charles VII, made the off-hand remark that "Charles VII is a good enough saint for me. He put 30,000 francs in my pocket when he brought the pox to France." Germany's Fugger family, the greatest bankers of the day, made a fortune as the chief importers of guaiacum, promoted as a cure for syphilis in Europe. In his book on syphilis, Gabriello Fallopius advised men to wash their genitals after sex, the first suggestion that European disregard for personal hygiene was a factor in the spread of the disease. For the most part, fear of syphilis or other diseases did not contribute to greatly improved hygiene, since most people did not know about the cause of disease until the end of the nineteenth century.

The disease was widespread among aristocrats, altering the political dynamics of many European countries. Friends of Lorenzo de Medici, Duke of Urbino, noticed he had boils and blisters on his legs when they helped him climb into his marriage bed. His wife died in childbirth, and he followed in 1519 when he was only twenty-seven years old. Britain's Tudors and France's Valois families were unable to bear living children, and uncertainty about succession fueled the period's civil wars. One or two of Mary Queen of Scots' husbands died of syphilis, suggesting she was infected as well. Italy's Borgia family was infected, and some thought Pope Julius II would not allow supplicants to kiss his feet because he too had the disease. By 1566 syphilis had incapacitated the Ottoman sultans of Turkey. Death and infertility in the aristocracy from syphilis created more room at the top, accelerating social mobility. Among commoners, the disease contributed to an overall slowdown in birth rates in Europe during the 1500s and 1600s, in the same way that it caused a decline in European birth rates at the end of the nineteenth century.

Syphilis also changed personal and social relationships because "fear of infection tended to erode the bonds of respect and trust that bound men and women together. The prostitute's chance of Christian forgiveness faded," historian Alfred Crosby said. In 1497 the town council of Aberdeen, Scotland, ordered that "all light women desist from their vice and sin of venery and work for their support, on pain, else, of being branded with a hot iron on their cheek and banished from the town." With Luther raging at "venemous syphilitic whores" who should be "broken on the wheel and flayed" for the harm they did to young men, syphilis was a boost to growing puritanical sentiments. In sixteenth and seventeenth century European Catholicism and Protestantism, they "could hardly have occurred without the fear that syphilis brought to sexuality," according to historian William McNeill. Puritanism would not have had such a wide appeal and gained adherents so quickly and widely without the threat of syphilis. The plague made many Europeans doubt the efficacy of religion, but syphilis did the Renaissance church in, ushering in a new interest in asceticism. "Never afterwards can we find brazenly licentious Popes (like the Borgias) or monasteries where open fornication was the rule," comments historian Stanislav Andreski.

Since people who obeyed religious strictures about monogamy were less likely to contract syphilis, self-protection encouraged decorum. Brothels and public baths were closed in the 1520s and 1530s, although the Catholic church's officially sanctioned brothels continued to operate until the Reformation took firm hold. Fewer cheeks were kissed in greeting, and people avoided casual contact of any kind. The Catholic church began to crack down on illicit sex in 1563. Antiprostitution campaigns were especially fierce in Toledo and Seville, and the Inquisition used harsh methods to reform wayward offenders. Sexual relationships were fraught not only with the possibility of syphilis but gonorrhea, changing the tenor of the romantic, loving interchanges of the Renaissance from trust to suspicion.

Survival favored "people of stern morals, who avoided fornication and adultery and who chose as spouses persons of similar conduct... libertines died young and left a few sickly dependents," according to Andreski. Protestantism linked success in commerce to prudent behaviors, including frugality, hard work, and saving. Abstinence fostered early capitalism, encouraging abhorrence of pleasures and dedication to work or contemplative self-mortification. Capitalism was further linked with the Calvinist doctrine of predestination, which viewed charity as unnecessary because the condition of all humans was preordained before their birth. This doctrine stimulated accumulation of capital because it provided an excuse for abandoning the old Christian commandment of charity. God had damned the poor and they deserved no alms.

By the mid-sixteenth century, the idea of celibacy before marriage began to take hold in Protestant and Catholic doctrine, and Watts says that "prostitutes were no longer seen as the flowers in the crown of a properly governed city as they had been in the early 1490s; instead they were regarded as petty criminals." Prostitution continued, however, because poor girls and women could earn money much more quickly than they could as domestics or in other more acceptable jobs, the same pattern that now encourages the spread of AIDS. Then as now, "male clientele was always on hand," says Watts. "Wherever soldiers were billeted, brothels were an easy way to keep them out of worse mischief." They also served the needs of rural men, who were more afraid of the consequences of masturbation than the chance of contracting syphilis.

To protect their soldiers and transit laborers, French authorities began registering prostitutes in cities with barracks in 1802. Male army medics inspected the women using the "state penis," or speculum. Although the rubber condom had been invented in England in the 1840s, few used them, believing (possibly because of Fallopius) that washing with water after intercourse would kill any germs. In the mid-1870s Alfred Fournier warned that "syphilis can, because of its consequences, debase and corrupt the species by producing inferior, decadent, dystrophic, and deficient beings," and, together with his son, warned women to look for specific physical markers showing syphilitic inheritance in a prospective husband's family, including hollowed-out upper incisor teeth. On both sides of the channel, the prostitute was believed to be "an atavistic throwback to earlier primitive human types with stronger arms and shoulders than normal women, deeper voices, and prehensile feet," Watts says. In debates over prostitution in the United States, repression won out over regulation because Progressives "refused to compromise with evil," says historian Alan Brandt. A new medical specialty, syphilogy, was created in the late 1800s, endowed with university chairs, national and international societies, and conferences.

Fear of venereal diseases became even more widespread after the severe systemic effects of syphilis and gonorrhea were documented in the mid- to late 1800s. But European physicians were still anxious to protect the confidentiality of their syphilitic clients, warning young men contemplating marriage to delay for four years until mercury treatment took effect but not to tell their beloveds that they had the disease. In the first decade of the twentieth century, English physicians decried German physician Iwan Bloch's suggestion that young people be properly educated and warned so they would not contract the disease. While some American physicians, including John Stokes of the Mayo Clinic, argued that failing to inform partners was a "blind policy of protecting the guilty at the expense of the innocent," most thought that keeping the patient's secret was in the interest of the social order. A self-administered mercuric compound was developed in the eighteenth century so that suffers could treat themselves and deceive their spouses.

Guy de Maupassant, believing that syphilitic madness would bring creativity to full flower, finally caught it and then deliberately gave it to Parisian prostitutes until he died, mad, in 1893. Flaubert did the same in Cairo. Only in Norway was conscious transmission of the disease a legal crime resulting in a jail sentence of three years, a practice Norwegian immigrants carried with them to the American state of Minnesota. Switzerland followed suit, but Britain, Italy, and Belgium relied on medical inspections of prostitutes to hold the line against the disease. Infecting someone with syphilis did not become a crime in Denmark, Sweden, Czechoslovakia, and the Soviet Union until after the World War I.

Like lepers in medieval Europe, prostitutes in Italy were consigned to "hospitals" where they were forced to work and pray and were punished with starvation if they had any contact with the outside world. Even victims of sexual violence were confined to asylums for "reeducation," so they could resist further sexual advances. Since most young men delayed marriage for economic reasons, physicians helped them avoid masturbation and seduction of "honest" women through the state's system of regulated prostitution. Prostitutes were viewed as having physical and moral characteristics that suited them for the trade, including frigidity, precocity, and "moral insanity," traits more common among young lower-class women from southern Italy. State regulation targeted the poor because prostitutes were almost exclusively poor women. They were placed under sanitary and police control, and poor men—conscript soldiers, criminals, and vagabonds—were also subject to compulsory medical inspection.

Masturbation had been encouraged until the end of the seventeenth century as a way to prepare a boy for marriage, and in the French court of Henry IV "the king's friends amused themselves by strengthening the manly organ of the infant dauphin," Watts says. In 1690 a Swiss minister, Jean Frederic Osterwald, capitalized on a growing anti-masturbation trend by describing its dreadful results, and quacks wandered from village to village selling "cures" for sexual urges. By 1756 a Swiss physician, S. Tissot, published a medical text to educate physicians on how to cure the disability, based on Hippocrates's idea that masturbation drained the richness of the blood by producing throw-away sperm. It also purportedly reduced memory, understanding, concentration, caused headaches, loss of appetite, bloody urine, and enfeebled the genitals. The enjoyment of both partners in heterosexual intercourse, by contrast, restored the blood system. Jean-Jacques Rousseau defined masturbation as unnatural sex and warned tutors to watch their students like hawks, tucking them in only when sleepy and raising them from bed the moment they were awake. A century later, in 1860, a man seeking treatment for syphilis wrote that his doctor had advised him to give up masturbation and visit prostitutes instead, even telling him where to find "certain houses where I might meet women of a better class."

Using arguments similar to those used in Africa by opponents of condom promotion for HIV/AIDS prevention, prominent American physicians argued against eradication of syphilis (even after the discovery of penicillin) because it would remove the last vestige of social control of immoral behavior. Johns Hopkins physician Howard Kelly stated that "if we could in an instant eradi-cate the diseases, we would also forget at once the moral side of the question, and would then, in one short generation, fall wholly under the domination of animal passions, becoming grossly and universally immoral." As syphilis raged, belief in the evils of masturbation became almost universal. In 1899 German medical specialist Hermann Rohledler published evidence that masturbation destroyed the central nervous system. Providers of sexual advice, such as Britain's Marie Stopes, received innumerable letters from men who could not stop the habit. One young man wrote that he had sex with different girls two to three nights a week before he was married to cure himself of the problem. Since this was typical of the bad medical advice given young men, syphilis flourished as never before, spread by men Sheldon Watts calls "terrified mas-turbators in search of a cure." In Italy and England, feminists argued against a double standard of behavior for males and females, but England's Social Purity movement castigated physicians for scaring young men so badly about the dan-gers of syphilis that they took up the "far more lethal sport of masturbation."

✳ ✳ ✳

In the late nineteenth century, controlling syphilis became even more urgent for western states dismayed at declines in fertility occurring just at a time when men were needed to build up armed forces for a European war. The search for a cure followed quickly after two German microbiologists,

Fritz Schaudinn and Eric Hoffmann, identified the cause of syphilis in 1905. The seriousness of the disease's prevalence is reflected in the fact that the first "Magic Bullet," or specific remedy, ever developed in biomedicine was for syphilis. The Wasserman test, developed in 1906, allowed positive diagnosis. In 1909 Paul Ehrlich, a disciple of Robert Koch, produced an effective compound, Salvarsan, on his 606th experiment with aniline dyes, and by 1912 he refined the drug into Neosalvarsan, which had fewer side effects. Sulpha drugs (sulfonamides) were also effective against gonorrhea.

Given prevailing social attitudes, syphilis and gonorrhea did not become what public health specialists call "reportable diseases" until well after World War I, but some idea of the size of the problem can be gained from military records. Almost 30 percent of American soldiers serving in the 1916 campaign against Mexico's Pancho Villa had venereal diseases, and in some camps, as many as 300 men applied for Salvarsan treatments every day. The level of venereal disease in American training camps for World War I, which included a broader range of recruits, was 13 percent in 1918. Between April 1917 and December 1919, 383,706 soldiers were diagnosed with syphilis, gonorrhea, or chancroid. During World War I, black American soldiers were reputed to have such high rates of syphilis that the mayor of St. Nazaire, France, asked that black women be brought over for their "use." In reality, the infection rate of white recruits was almost as high (32 per 1,000 among whites compared to 35.7 per 1,000 among blacks). In France, the prevailing rate in the general population at the time of the war was about 10 percent.

STD prevention among American soldiers was stymied by the American Social Hygiene Association, which fought hard to prohibit condom use in the early 1900s. In the minds of Association members, anyone who risked getting an STD deserved the consequences. The "dough boys"—U.S. soldiers who fought in World War I—were the only armed forces in Europe during the war who were denied the use of condoms. The Progressive Movement placed responsibility at the individual's doorstep, making "anti-venereal exhortations" to the troops demanding "*self*-discipline, *self*-denial, *self*-sacrifice, and *self*-control," according to Brandt. Education campaigns tried to frighten soldiers into changing their sexual behavior, but wartime conditions loosened social restraints. By September 1919, 766 of every 1,000 American soldiers stationed in France had an STD. Only the U.S. Navy was spared. Although his boss, the secretary of the U.S. Navy, believed condoms immoral and un-Christian, Franklin Delano Roosevelt, then assistant secretary of the Navy (and later U.S. president), ordered the distribution of prophylactic kits containing Salvarsan to sailors to treat the STDs they could have avoided with the condoms they were not allowed to use.

Syphilis gained an enormous boost after World War I, when soldiers returning to their homelands from the battlefields of Europe carried the disease around the world one more time. Soldiers from as far distant as Memphis and Atlanta, Sydney and Auckland, Johannesburg and Durban, Abidjan and Dakar, Nairobi and Entebbe, New York and St. Louis brought back memories of warm welcomes in European cities that extended beyond bonbons and freshly baked bread. But behavior that had been tolerated during wartime horrified their wives and sweethearts—and public health specialists—who were afraid the returning soldiers' families would be infected with syphilis. In France, Britain, and the United States, the public was "obsessed with syphilis and its dangers, concentrated on preaching abstinence and otherwise retreating in shame before sexual openness," says historian Jo Hays. By 1918 new laws passed in thirty-two states required compulsory detention and examination of prostitutes. High rates of rejection of military recruits with venereal diseases between the two world wars led to the establishment of a state-level public health surveillance system. During the 1930s, public demand grew in the United States for a national campaign against STDs, stimulated by a *Reader's Digest* article entitled "Why Don't We Stamp Out Syphilis?" Concern was economic as well. Treatment of venereal diseases during World War I had cost the U.S. government almost $50 million, says Brandt.

World War I created an especially serious health crisis for black American soldiers and their families. Syphilis rates among black and white American soldiers during World War I had been about equal, but rates among blacks soared to 252.3 per 1,000 by 1941, while rates among whites dropped to 17.4 per 1,000 from their World War I levels. The death rate for white men from syphilis increased to 28 per 100,000, but it was more than three times higher among black men (98 per 100,000). Infection rates for white and black women were 9 and 41 per thousand respectively. Between the wars, blacks were much less likely to seek treatment because of economic and cultural barriers. When they did seek treatment, it was from public clinics that were more likely to report the results to public health authorities. Tuberculosis levels during the same period were at epidemic levels, and heart disease rates were also much higher among blacks, differentials that persist today.

In 1932 U.S. Public Health Service experts initiated a study of the effects of untreated syphilis on black men in the United States as part of League of Nations' multicountry research. The Tuskegee Study withheld treatment from 400 men to see how syphilis progressed, even after it became known that penicillin could cure the disease. The men's health had already deteriorated badly because they were being treated with mercury rubs at the time the research began. The study's official reports are shocking, describing the terrible impact of late-stage syphilis on the men and their families in neutral and high-minded scientific language. Treatment was withheld from the men and their families even when the enormous systemic damage they sustained led to high death rates. The study was only called to a halt after a *New York Times* reporter exposed its chilling details in 1972.

❊ ❊ ❊

It has long been assumed that the extermination of Native Americans was due to European diseases such as typhus and smallpox, but the evidence for this is largely impressionistic, collected by soldiers, missionaries, trappers, and traders. In most parts of the Americas, it is difficult to document how many people were there originally, how many died, and how many were run off or absorbed into other tribes. To historian Alfred Crosby, Hawaii is a "controlled study," like the Darwin's Galapagos, because the population is confined and more reliable statistics are available. When Captain James Cook arrived in 1778, he counted 242,000 Hawaiian Polynesians, although demographers now estimate there were actually about 800,000 native residents on the island. In just over 100 years, only 48,000 were left. Only the import of Chinese workers starting in the 1850s, followed by immigration of Japanese, Philippine, and Portuguese laborers, "saved the Islands from the kind of demographic and economic decline that afflicted sixteenth-century Mexico," Crosby says. Even when the total population started to rise after 1878, the number of native Hawaiians continued to decline until the twentieth century.

Crosby's careful study of the data suggests a startling conclusion. Death rates soared, but birth rates also declined, due to "infanticide by neglect" and venereal disease, which reduced fertility. STDs were common among nearly all classes of Hawaiians, whom Crosby describes as a "sexually exploited population with a lethally obsolete set of sexual mores." His thesis is supported by a 1895 report from the American Bureau of Indian Affairs comparing two groups of tribes, four with limited European contact that were chaste, had no venereal disease, and were increasing in number; and seven with continuous contact, promiscuity, and widespread venereal disease that had steadily declining populations, diminishing 43 percent between 1882 and 1895. An eighteenth century missionary, John Heckewelder, noted that Amerindians varied in their attitudes, and while some tribes were not infected, many were "greatly infected" with venereal diseases.

What Crosby says is a "correlation between the restrictive or liberal attitudes toward sexuality of various groups and their survival or extinction" is also supported by other travelers' reports. In the Chinook tribes encountered by Meriwether Lewis, a young woman commonly offered her body because "her person is, in fact, often the only property of the young female, and is therefore the medium of trade, the return for presents, and the reward for service." Traders often came to the Chinook, so Lewis's companions were not the first white men these women had seen, and they had already developed coping strategies. Captain John Smith's description of his reception by the women of Powhatan and the probable results were similar. "Europe was in the midst of a pandemic of syphilis in this era, and if Smith did not carry the infection, it is likely that several of his comrades did," Crosby believes. The Virginian natives suffered epidemics over the next two centuries on the scale of those suffered by the Hawaiians. Thomas Jefferson, countering a remark by the Comte de Buffon that Native American Indians had small genitalia and a meager sex drive, said they had plenty of sex drive but few offspring, which he blamed on birth control, abortion, hunger, and overexertion. To Crosby, "an examination of the Hawaiian experience suggests a broader and even grimmer interpretation." Infertility was rampant, resulting from "the secret blights of abortion, infanticide and infanticidally negligent child care, venereal infection, sterility, and despair."

✖ ✖ ✖

By the mid-1860s British Contagious Disease (CD) Acts were consolidated within a broader "national-imperial policy," and by 1870 laws governing the control of contagious diseases, including STDs, were in place in British colonies and in all treaty ports where the country had interests. Colonial legislation was more stringent than domestic and covered more of the civilian population than British law. The acts emphasized "risk populations," which included the poor and women. Clients—men who used poor women's bodies for sexual outlet—were never mentioned, much as they are neglected in public health regulations and programs to prevent HIV transmission in developing countries today. In Vietnam, like many countries, sex work is a "social evil" punishable with incarceration, fines, and reeducation, but use of a sex worker by a man is not.

Laws in the colonies had to be much tougher than at home because "primitive" practices required harsher enforcement. In arguing for passage of a tough law in Hong Kong, a British administrative officer claimed that three-quarters of Chinese women were sex workers and exaggerated the extent and brutality of "Chinese sexual slavery." While STD rates were very high in Hong Kong, Shanghai, and Singapore—fueled by informal sex work by poor women, sexual slavery, and concubines, many of whom had hereditary syphilis—his overstatement was symptomatic of British views. Hong Kong was the center of an Asian flesh market, which then, as now, entangled women who had no other means of survival. Prostitution was big business, and women could be bought for between $150 and $500 at the beginning of the twentieth century, depending on their virginity, age, beauty, and ethnic origin. The same conditions prevailed in colonial Malaya, which was part of an international sex trade that trafficked in women and children. The trade capitalized growth of legitimate businesses in Penang, which at the turn of the twentieth century had over 100 brothels along Campbell Street named after towns in China. It also flourished in Manila, where STDs and sex work were common, serving soldiers, sailors, and foreigners with money to spend. A special hospital was established in Manila in 1740 for Spanish soldiers convalescing from STDs, and in 1766 syphilis was so common among prominent families that its victims married with no hesitation and the disease became an "inheritance" of which few families were free.

The Victorians thought that tropical climates acted as breeding grounds for disease, inflamed passions, and negated reason. Sex workers affronted their idea of women as "guardians of the sanitized home and sanctified hearth," and in a world where "cleanliness was next to Godliness," hygiene and femininity were linked in what some cynics have called the "soap saga" of Britain's evolutionary superiority. Primitive peoples, they believed, were simply more tolerant of filth and STDs because of their unrestrained sexuality, both symptoms of nonwestern moral decay. In the 1860s, however, STDs were rampant among returning soldiers and in British garrisons overseas, suggesting that moral decay was infectious and stringent measures of control were badly needed.

The Victorian view of Africa was highly charged with images of violence and heroism, contrasting the "primitive" and "civilized" states of humankind according to the new theories of evolution. Political elites boldly manipulated the idea of "white man's burden" to gain public support for their conquests. Only King Leopold of Belgium's strategies in the Congo came up for public criticism because they were a particularly cynical example of abuse and manipulation, but other powers also recognized the necessity of manipulating public support for their noble interests while sustaining behind-the-scenes rape of their colonial possessions.

In the Victorian era's scrambled notions of sexuality, "primitive" humans were thought to have wildly different sexual habits and behavior than their "cultivated" European contemporaries. To some European colonialists, African sexuality was especially dark, primitive, uncontrolled, and excessive, epitomizing the dangers of the "Dark Continent." For others, it was essentially innocent, but had degenerated as a result of colonial contact. Christianity had destroyed indigenous moral systems, displacing traditionally severe punishments for sexual offenses, and had not replaced them with other systems of social control. Colonial administrators were reluctant to interfere in the conduct of sexual relations, but the Eugenics movement growing out of Darwin's theory of evolution created interest in genetically engineering "improved" populations that could more easily bear colonial labor demands.

In a 1908 debate in the *Lancet* and the *British Medical Journal* over the causes of syphilis, scientists suggested for the first time that disease could worsen because of colonial contact. Some authorities claimed that 80 percent of the population of Africa had syphilis, increasing the infant mortality rate to 50 to 60 percent. In Uganda, rates of syphilis were so high that many believed the Baganda, Uganda's largest tribe, were a "dying race." At the prompting of the British, their chiefs made treatment compulsory in 1913 and donated their subjects' tribute labor to build Mulago Hospital, complete with isolation wards for higher-class syphilis patients. Among some Baganda, syphilis became fashionable, because the British had focused attention on the plight of these aristocrats and the depopulation of their rich country. Buganda and Bunyoro men were eager to be treated, but women, subjected to compulsory physical exams, were not.

Missionaries joined with the colonial government to wage an all-out Uganda Venereal Disease Campaign in the early 1920s, which the Baganda elite supported to reestablish some of the control they had lost over younger men and women during the early colonial period. By the early 1920s British medical officers realized that they may have been misdiagnosing yaws and "native syphilis" as venereal syphilis, and by 1938 reported cases of yaws and syphilis shifted in importance. Historians later learned that not only were yaws and syphilis confused in early diagnoses, but endemic, nonvenereal syphilis had been confused with both yaws and venereal syphilis because they were all caused by the same spirochetes. With treatment, endemic syphilis declined rapidly in the first half of the century, replaced by venereal syphilis, a much more severe, intractable, and resistant disease. This trend was also reported in other African territories.

The British secretary of state for the colonies sent a circular to the governors of his African territories in 1930 noting that the empire's African subjects were not "reproducing themselves at a sufficient rate to ensure the economic viability of the colonies." Missionary and philanthropic organizations argued that the social pathology inherent in traditional customs was the cause. Nutritionists and anthropologists, on the other hand, blamed poverty, not social traditions. Colonial authorities decided that more information on "primitive customs" was needed, and in 1925 medical officers in Nyasaland (Malawi) were asked to report any practices or diseases that reduced native birth rates. Officers in migrant labor areas in northern Malawi reported that the absence of males and increase of STDs reduced the number of pregnancies and caused widespread spontaneous abortion and infertility. An Indian physician imported by the British to serve as medical director in the Fort Manning district went further, attributing low birth rates to "agricultural distress and the poverty of the masses." He advocated new cotton varieties and spinning technology to start rural industries that would alleviate poverty. In Northern Rhodesia (Zambia), reports from the late 1920s linked low birth rates to labor migration, but colonial officials argued that work in the mines improved male health status and physiques.

Women bore the brunt of the blame in this reproductive crisis for their poor infant and child feeding practices, and their infertility was viewed as a sign of their degeneration. But while the mother and child welfare movement tried to suppress female sexuality, in migrant labor areas, colonial administrators believed that African male sexuality required "expression" so it would not turn into dangerous rebellion, and African women were brought in to supply sexual services for male workers. Colonial governments tried to address the migrant labor system's disruption of marriage and kinship practices by bolstering marriage through customary courts, where the "women problem" was shorthand for problems of property rights, labor, and intergenerational relations.

Victorians believed that all females were inherently primitive and childlike, similar to "savages" in the territories. Medicine cooperated by finding that white female skulls resemble those of the "Negro." Medical Social Darwinists believed that differences between the sexes were less marked in "primitive peoples," including sexual characteristics. Victorians claimed that "women from the 'primitive races' were less differentiated from their men than were women in 'advanced' societies. Sexual differences became more marked as one moved up the evolutionary ladder," says historian Megan Vaughn. "Specific attention was given to the 'primitiveness' of the black woman's genitalia, and to her supposedly equally 'primitive' and powerful sexual appetite." But real African women were almost invisible to colonial medical services that concentrated on determining male fitness for work until after World War II. Colonial doctors, charged with maintaining large and productive labor forces, became concerned only when women's birth rates declined from infertility. Victorian missionaries, on the other hand, had always viewed African women as the repository of the evil and dark side of African culture because of their natural attitudes toward sexuality.

With World War II, reported cases of syphilis and gonorrhea increased, caused by recruitment, troop movements, and the general disruption of normal life. By 1944 STDs rose significantly in Kenya, and the black market in penicillin exploded. Wartime surges in syphilis and gonorrhea were reported in Uganda, Zambia, Zimbabwe, Tanzania, and Malawi. Military authorities targeted the "native prostitute" as the source of the problem, defended the reputation of their soldiers, and instituted enforced examination of women. But Dr. W. A. Young, the East African Command venereologist, argued that STDs were already epidemic in the army and feared a widespread and intractable general epidemic after the war. "We are preparing," he said, "a cornucopia for distribution among the homes of Africa, and are even now spilling ripe seeds as men go home on leave.'" New varieties of STDs made diagnosis and treatment more difficult and increased drug resistance. Due to the severity of the situation, Young argued that public health had to take priority over individual liberties to prevent rapid spread. Mission hospitals, following their own doctrines, charged more for treatment to discourage promiscuity. In one Nyasaland hospital, the payments financed the leper colony, but far fewer STD sufferers came for treatment.

While some directors of the British Colonial Medical Services favored funding to make diagnostic and treatment facilities more widely available and opposed restraint, control, and increased legal powers, others argued for a reform of African sexuality. H. S. deBoer, director of medical services for Uganda, believed that "the local African is especially immoral or even that he is amoral but that his way of looking at sexual contact is different from what is generally accepted to be that of the European Christian civilization." In his testimony before the medical committee, he argued that the war had worsened the disruption of native custom and social practice initiated by colonization. Since tradition could not be restored, a new morality had to be forged. He chafed against missionary influence, because there was a "time lag between the destruction of an indigenous moral code and the growth of a Christian code to replace it." One member of the committee remarked that "the only propaganda that was worthwhile was quick and free treatment... when enough of the population had been treated, V.D. would disappear," a technocrat's view opposed by committee members who feared that Christian morality would be undermined. The medical services directors told the committee that Africans attached little shame to STDs, which made treatment easier and legislation to control their spread unnecessary. The lack of funds to provide a widely available service embarrassed some medical officers, but others argued that Africans needed to learn a sense of shame. They said that even prominent African clergymen were known to be infected, and once

Africans saw that STDs could be treated, they would become even more promiscuous.

✳ ✳ ✳

According to human sexuality expert Anne Fausto-Sterling, our ideas of sexuality are rich and complex, but "we can not understand the origins of human sexual expression without knowing more about how we actually behave." Sexology, the study of human sexual behavior, began in the 1940s. Alfred Kinsey, Wardell Pomeroy, and Clyde Martin published the first scientific survey of behavior in 1948. Kinsey and his colleagues had discovered "a continuum of sexuality," on which they placed the reported "hetero" and "homo" sexual behavior reported in their survey. Over 37 percent of the men in their national sample reported overt homosexual experiences. Most occurred during adolescence, but 25 percent of the males had had "more than incidental homosexual experiences" for at least three years of their lives.

The book went through nine reprintings in the first year and a half because the public was hungry to know more about a taboo subject. The medical profession felt differently. The American Medical Association accused Kinsey of instigating "a wave of sex hysteria" in 1954, and Kinsey fell prey to the conservative backlash in the U.S. Congress, which accused him of causing "the depravity of a whole generation" and increasing juvenile delinquency. Pressured by the House committee that controlled tax-exempt status, the Rockefeller Foundation withdrew its support of Kinsey and he died in 1956, crushed by the vilification of his work. Kinsey met the same fate as pioneer English sexologist Havelock Ellis, who studied sexual behavior at the turn of the twentieth century. When Ellis's neutral, scientific treatment of homosexuality came out in 1897, his publisher faced criminal prosecution for the "lewd, wicked, bawdy, scandalous, and obscene" book. In Germany, Magnus Hirschfield's Institute for Study of Sexual Behavior, founded in 1919, started discussion groups, and by the 1930s more than 80 clinics had been opened to offer laypeople more information. In 1933, only months after their rise to power, the Nazis burned all the institute's books and papers and banned the talk groups.

In the early 1990s, U.S. congressmen withdrew funding for the first national study of sexual behavior in the United States since Kinsey's, even though the National Research Council warned in 1989 that "we don't know enough to win the war against sexually transmitted diseases, including AIDS." It argued that more information was desperately needed about sexual behavior and the relationship between sex and drug and alcohol use, espe-

cially among young people. It advocated longitudinal studies, especially of
teens, and its projects were just starting when funding was squelched. The
National Institute of Child Health and Development awarded a contract for
a Kinsey update to Edward Laumann, dean of the Division of Social Sciences
at the University of Chicago, who planned to study the influence of sexual
networks on behavior. He argued that the information gained from the study
would be instrumental in understanding the spread of STDs in different age
groups, but when U.S. Senator Jesse Helms, a notoriously conservative
Republican from North Carolina, learned about it, funding was immediately
withdrawn. Helms also pulled funding from a survey of teens and their parents at the University of North Carolina's Population Center one year after it
had been initiated, so the money could be put into organizations that
encouraged premarital celibacy. Surveys were canceled even though they were
supported by a broad cross-section of the American scientific community.
Detractors said they were part of a conspiracy by homosexuals in the
Department of Health and Human Services who want to legitimize homosexual life styles. "As long as I stand on the floor of the U.S. Senate," Helms
said, "I am never going to yield to that sort of thing because it is not just
another lifestyle, it is sodomy."

And now we find ourselves in the middle of a raging global AIDS epidemic
with very little information about how humans behave as sexual creatures.
One reason for suppression of wider sexual knowledge is, of course, the belief
that this knowledge increases sexual behavior, although study after study
demonstrates that knowledge counteracts impulsiveness and compulsiveness.
Teens armed with the facts tend to be much more responsible about their
choices. Keeping disease prevention information secret when pornographic
materials and sex in television and films abound is nothing but hypocritical.

Lack of real information also continues to feed the persistent belief that
"primitive Africans" have sexual behaviors vastly different from "civilized"
people. Molly's story shows us just how intrusive and unhelpful this attitude
is in shaping epidemic responses. Early research into AIDS in Africa helped
perpetuate the notion that African sexuality is bizarre and uncontrolled by
focusing on "ethnopornographic" details like dry sex and intercourse with
virgins and children. African commentators reversed the tables and argued
that AIDS is associated with the "perverse" western practice of homosexuality. As the epidemic has progressed, both sides have moved to the center,
pushing the wider framework of poverty that fuels the spread of HIV to the
foreground.

Physicians all over the world still find it difficult to initiate constructive
conversations with their patients about sexual behavior. So many STDs,

including HIV, remain hidden until they have caused extensive organ damage, infertility, and chronic disease. The incidence of STDs is astounding given their effects—human papillomavirus affects close to 50 percent of Americans and causes cancer—but not surprising given the heavy veil of secrecy, misinformation, and shame that we choose to drape over the subject of sex. In the end, serious diseases go undetected and unreported because of shame, and sexuality gets channeled into violent and exploitive expression, driven underground by shame. The same prejudices and fear that hindered responses to STDs throughout history continue to hamper our responses to HIV/AIDS in the world. The result? Unimpeded, frightening growth of the disease in country after country and the buildup of an enormous disease reservoir that mocks our prudishness and threatens our survival.

Darwin was sophisticated enough to realize that all human groups have basic similarities and are connected to African ancestors through their evolutionary origins, and he understood from his travels the dimensions of poverty and exploitation that characterized nineteenth-century colonialism. But the influence of Victorian sexual morality was so pervasive that it blinded this otherwise brilliant man to the one of the most important engines of human evolution, STDs, a disease threat that has shaped world history since the sixteenth century. In the same way, cultural inhibitions blind us to the reality of sexual drives and activities, their force in evolution, and their role in the transmission of disease. Knowing more about sexual behavior can help us understand how STDs actually spread and what drives the various expressions of human sexuality, essential parts of our armamentarium if we are to survive our contest with our microbes. With AIDS these killers have evolved the ultimate competitor for the welfare of human kind, and our ignorance could be our ultimate loss.

One positive aspect about this epidemic is that it is finally bringing us out of the closet to acknowledge the diversity of human sexual expression, its fluidity, its naturalness. We have seen how closely sexuality and disease are linked in shaping world history. HIV/AIDS is also revealing the ties of sexuality to greed and power, particularly as it plays itself out in gender relations. In the next chapter we will look at the evolutionary origins of sexuality to tie gender relations, sexuality, and disease together in another even more fundamental way.

CHAPTER SEVEN

Disease and Evolution

Dust raised by the departure of Save the Children and AIDS Control Program vehicles lingered in the air. Molly held her handkerchief over her mouth as she watched them disappear over the hill, racing to get back to Kampala before nightfall. As she turned toward Robina and Pauline, she wiped her face so they would not see her tears. The two women were sitting on the wall of the verandah, and Pauline's long, thin frame seemed to have collapsed onto itself. Robina fanned herself distractedly with a sheaf of papers from the orphan count, and Molly scurried to recapture one that had broken loose and drifted in the soft breeze. The chiefs had scattered, climbing on their bicycles or walking to the taxi park. A few had caught a ride with Save the Children to Masaka and would continue to more distant parts of the district from there. Another meeting where lots had been said but nothing had been resolved.

The British had heard it all: the starving, unkempt children, AIDS victims dying without care or medicine, the fear and panic being experienced by the district's residents, and the chiefs' commitment to action on the programs initiated by Robina, Molly, and Pauline. There was simply nothing more that could be done or said to convince them of the need to start programs on a wide scale immediately. The AIDS Control Program staff had averted their eyes when the discussion of budgets started. They had money, Molly knew, but not nearly enough to conduct even modest prevention programs around the country, which was their first priority.

Well, Molly thought cheerfully, maybe the box they brought had some blankets. She pulled it out onto the veranda then sat back on her heels and sighed. "Nothing but condoms," she said, more to herself than to the two women.

"And not enough of those, either," Pauline grumbled. "Let's not waste any more time here," Robina said, standing suddenly. She dusted off her skirt and started down the stairs. "I want you two in my office in half an hour. Once you make sure everything's cleared away, come right down." Pauline watched her figure recede through squinted eyes and then looked at Molly with a sour expression. "Wonder what she's up to now." Molly smiled. "I'm not going to be late to find out. Let's get this place cleaned up and go down there."

"Did you hear all that talk about male circumcision?" Pauline grinned. "I thought Wallace would just die, and the reverend looked like he'd been bitten by a large dog in the wrong place!" "It makes sense," Molly countered. "They said Muslim men don't get the infection as easily because of it. I supposed if you can wash properly, you'd get rid of some of the germs." "If these people had more water to wash with, there'd be fewer germs of any kind," Pauline replied. "Half the women I visit spend most of their day hauling water. Most of it's runoff water, and the way they reuse it they probably spread more germs than they kill."

"Mrs. Kategera's children didn't look like they'd bathed in a week when I was over there the other day," Molly agreed. "The barrel they had to collect rainwater had rotted through, so I had to haul water myself to wash them and their clothes. I asked a couple of the chiefs today if they could find some relatives to take the children when their mother dies. If not, I'll have to add them to that little house I started for the other orphans, but there's not much more room. After I dressed them the other day, they asked me to walk down to their father's grave with them." She blinked. "It's a terrible thing to think that pretty soon their mother will be lying under another heap of dirt in that little banana grove. Two little sticks tied with string was the only cross marking their father's grave, and as we stood there, the poor little things held my hands so tight I started to cry right along with them."

"At least our children are nearly grown," Pauline said, putting her arm around Molly's shoulder. "Come on now. We've done all we can here. Let's see what Robina's got on her mind." Robina's secretary was typing furiously on the little manual when they came through the door. Robina gestured at her. "I'm sending a letter to all the chiefs," she explained, "asking them to start organizing committees in their villages. Tomorrow I'm going to go see Abdul Rasheed."

"Do you think he's circumcised?" Pauline interrupted, and they all giggled. "It's a good thing you never lose your sense of humor, Pauline," Robina said, wiping her eyes. "No, that's not what I'm going down there to find out. I want to see how he's organizing his villages, and I want you two to come with me." Pauline perked up. "Let's get him to go to other chiefs and help them get started." "Exactly what I thought we should do," Robina nodded. "Molly, I want you to identify some of the women you've been working with who are setting up day care centers and communal gardens who could go to other villages and tell them how it works."

"I was wondering," Pauline began. "I know I shouldn't try to tell people who are inspired by God how to do things, but do you think the missionaries my son is working for could help? They probably need a project to keep them out of mischief." "The reverend asked me if he might organize the church women into a club," Molly said excitedly, "because he thinks they could help make blankets and start to bring in some used clothes from the Kampala dioceses." "A lot of families need soap, toothbrushes, small things like that," Robina said. "I could ask some of the merchants in town to donate a few items a month. I think most of them would help." The secretary had stopped typing. "You know, my husband's part of the farmers' cooperative," she said. "Maybe they could use that old tractor to plow up some more fields for matooke and ground nuts and greens." They were talking so loudly that no one heard the truck pull up. The tall, dark haired woman stood at the door with her hands on her hips and cleared her throat.

"Mrs. Nyeko?" Robina came forward. "I'm Donatella Lorch, a reporter with the *New York Times*."[1]

⚹ ⚹ ⚹

In his travels around the world, Darwin encountered the worst human misery he had ever seen, caused by the oppressive conditions of colonial labor. From the copper mines in Quillota, Chile, he reported that "the laboring men work very hard [and] with twelve pounds per annum, they have to clothe themselves and support their families." At an American gold mine in Chile Darwin saw men carrying ore 450 feet up ladders to the surface. Each man carried 200 pounds on his back, "quite naked excepting drawers," pale, poor and kept alive on boiled beans and bread. "They would prefer having bread alone; but their masters, finding that they cannot work so hard on this, treat them like horses, and make them eat the beans." Agricultural laborers fared worse. Darwin was pleased to meet a family of "pure Indian extraction" in the Andes, "aborigines advanced to the same degree of civilization, however low that may be, which their white conquerors have attained." Chile's 1832 census showed only 11,000 inhabitants with Indian surnames, "not all of pure breed," survivors of a Spanish Inquisition at Lima that had purged all the Indians still practicing pre-Columbian religious rites.

In his *Journals* Darwin ranked the humans he saw on a continuum. Tierra del Fuegians from the toe of South America existed "in a lower state of improvement than in any other part of the world." The inhabitants of Otaheite (Tahiti), governed by hereditary kings, were far higher on Darwin's social scale than the Maori of New Zealand, who practiced polygamy and kept slaves. Like the women, they could be executed summarily if they displeased their masters. Although he never saw them, he believed that the "Esquimau" were as "civilized" as South Sea Islanders, who were not only physically beautiful, but had "a mildness in the expression of their countenances which at once banishes the idea of a savage; and an intelligence which shows that they are advancing in civilization." The *Beagle*'s crew joined the Tahitians in a bonfire-lit songfest, and, while trading with them the next day, Darwin was surprised to learn that they "now fully understand the value of money, and prefer it to old clothes or other articles" because they wanted to buy boats and horses. Unfortunately, Darwin said, the women were physically unattractive, considerably less "moral" than the men.

The Malay slaves of Keeling Island in the Indian Ocean were so superstitious they believed in the power of a dancing "spoon," and South African tribesmen, "prowling about in search of roots, and living concealed on the wild and arid plains, are [also] sufficiently wretched." In Darwin's opinion, only Australian Aborigines were as savage as the Fuegians. When he visited Australia, the Aboriginal population was in decline. The introduction of alcohol and European diseases and the extinction of wild animals were responsible, Darwin wrote. "Even the milder [diseases], such as the measles, prove very destructive, and "numbers of their children invariably perish in very early infancy from the effects of their wandering life." Colonial settlers had taken their richest land, and "as the difficulty of procuring food increases, so must their wandering habits increase." To Darwin it was "remarkable how the same disease is modified in different climates. At the little island of St. Helena the introduction of scarlet fever is dread as a plague. In some countries, foreigners and natives are as differently affected by certain contagious disorders as if they had been different animals."

No human fossils had yet been found that could help Darwin decide where humans originated, and he told Wallace that in *The Origin of the Species*, he would "avoid the whole subject, as so surrounded with prejudices, though I fully admit that it is the highest and most interesting problem for the naturalist." After examining chimps and gorillas brought back by explorers from Africa, Thomas Huxley and other biologists concluded that they were closer to humans than to the orangutan. The connection between humans and apes was difficult to believe because humans had much more powerful brains; even Wallace concluded that divine intervention was responsible for that final transformation. Darwin knew that humans and great apes were virtually identical in their embryonic development and changed proportions only very late in embryonic growth. These similarities were so convincing that he ignored Wallace's opinion and the discovery of a Neanderthal fossil and early human tools in Europe in 1856. Readers of his *Descent of Man* learned that "it is somewhat more probable that our early progenitors lived on the African continent than elsewhere."

✳ ✳ ✳

However much advocates of the "multiregion" and "African origin" theories of evolution may disagree about when the first humans left Africa, they do agree that the first creature we recognize as human evolved on the high grasslands and wooded slopes of eastern and southern Africa. Ever since Darwin first suggested that the human species was born in Africa, conclusive genetic evidence has been piling up, supporting a growing body of fossil evidence unavailable when Darwin first made the suggestion. Genetic evidence now shows that every living person descended from a relatively small group of Africans who lived between 100,000 and 200,000 years ago. It is not an accident of archaeology or geology that all significant proto- and early human fossils have been found in Africa, because all the major events in human evolution occurred there.

Five million years ago, climatic change prompted the last common ancestor of humans and chimps to drop from the trees and spend more time living on the African savannah. Four million years ago, the proto-humans began spending most of their time on their feet, and 2 million years after that began altering natural objects to use as tools, finally mastering fire about 500,000 years ago. When the first recognizably modern humans evolved around 150,000 years ago, they numbered several tens of thousands and were surrounded by more than a million archaic proto-humans. There were at least four different types of hominids alive at the time, all adapted to slightly different econiches. New species can form in the middle of an existing species' range because the center of the range is where resources are greatest and foster population growth. Dense populations provide rich genetic diversity on which evolution can act. They are "genetic hot spots" where new variations arise. Humans emerged into very tumultuous times when the global climate was rapidly cooling, turning sub-Saharan Africa's jungles into patches of woodland and savannah. While the chimps clung to the forests, humans adapted to the open habitat of the grasslands, losing their fingerlike toes and evolving longer legs. Heads and backs were held more upright as our first ancestors learned to walk on two feet, picking fruit off low-hanging branches and improving their hunting skills.

Although coexisting groups of modern and archaic humans seem to have lived peacefully, intergroup competition probably provided the impetus for modern humans to migrate to other continents. In the first wave, *Homo erectus*, the direct ancestor of modern humans (*Homo sapiens*), reached Asia 1.8 to 1.6 million years ago, and Neanderthals reached the Middle East and Europe by 150,000 years ago. Advocates of the multiregional theory of evolution believe that was the last migration from African, and that modern humans evolved in many different parts of Asia and Europe from *Homo erectus* ancestors. However, more recent genetic analyses have erased all doubts that there was a second wave of migration starting about 100,000 years ago. According to the African origin theory of evolution, in the second wave, migrating *Homo sapiens* moved north along the Nile Valley, across the Sinai peninsula, and into the Fertile Crescent and Europe between 51,000 and 39,000 years ago. By 60,000 years ago, modern humans had found their way to the coastal sections of India and Southeast Asia. They sailed to Australia 50,000 years ago, crossing the shallow seas that separated it from Asia, and by 12,000 years ago, they had migrated north, crossed the land bridge joining Siberia and Alaska, and spread south to populate North and South America.

Early human hunters and gatherers, searching constantly for new food sources, migrated faster and farther than groups of *Homo erectus* had because their technology was superior. They occupied all the continents except Antarctica within 50,000 years after they left Africa, displacing their archaic relatives everywhere the two came into contact. Modern humans did not interbreed with older species, nor did they fight; *Homo sapiens* was simply a superior hunter and bred faster. The genetic lineage of all modern humans is known as L3 and is one of the three African "daughters of Eve." Every human alive can trace his or her genetic family tree to one of these three daughters or to one of the five Asian daughters, four American daughters, or seven European daughters. While these migrating groups spent enough time apart to establish themselves as clear genetic lines (what used to be called races), they began to come back into contact with one another as populations got larger. Like any varieties, they mated and swapped genes, and any differences among the populations blended away. Human groups never "speciated," that is, they never remained apart long enough to reach the point where they could no longer breed together, becoming separate species.

Because only one of the African "Eves" migrated from the continent to become the mother of all other genetic lines, modern humans cluster into two distinct groups based on DNA similarity. One group includes modern Africans, and the other includes everyone else, so the "populations outside of Africa are closer genetically to each other than they are to populations within Africa," says evolutionary biologist John Relethford. This difference may provide some deep explanation of indifference to Africa's condition on the part of most other human groups. Although this explanation may be tantalizing, it is probably best left at the back of the philosophical shelf, because most of the physical markers that define "Africans" are nothing more than environmental adaptations and are shared by many other human groups on the planet.

In the end, we all trace our ultimate genetic heritage back to our African roots. Genetic studies of living humans have determined that the Bushmen of southern Africa, now living primarily in Botswana, were one of the earliest distinct populations to appear after modern humans evolved, and they have the oldest traceable genetic material of any group in the world.[2] According to geneticist Himla Soodyall, "the basis of our genetic diversity was established ... in Africa. At some point a group of people who carried just a subset of that diversity left Africa, and they gave rise to all the populations that we see today outside of Africa." Their superior antiquity explains why Africans have the greatest genetic diversity of any human group alive today. Until a population explosion some 60,000 to 100,000 years ago forced groups to spread out to other continents, the majority of humans lived in Africa, Relethford says, and it was the most densely populated landmass in the world. Relethford speaks for all evolutionary biologists when he says that the traditional concept of human "race" is useless because genetic analysis has found that all humans overlap so much that the genetic difference *between* "races" is smaller than the difference *within* "races." A number of large-scale comparative studies of human genetic material since 1972 show on average that 90 percent of the variation in humans occurs within "races" and only 10 percent between. Traditional markers of "racial" difference, such as skin color, facial characteristics, and hair type are shared among races. High levels of gene flow among human populations makes it almost impossible to establish clear-cut boundaries among different groups of people.

Nevertheless, diversity—or variation, as biologists call it—is wide in the human species because of environmental pressures, many of which are exerted through diseases. Some traits, such as skin color, vary across smooth gradients, while others vary in small pockets in response to specific environmental conditions. Skin color is darkest at the equator, lightens gradually as one moves toward the poles, and is darker overall in the southern hemisphere than in the northern. Differences in skin color correspond to the amount of ultraviolet radiation received at any given location on the earth's surface. That amount is highest at the equator, so the risk of burning and skin cancer, which increases with sun exposure, is higher there. Darker-skinned people have a higher concentration of melanin near the skin's surface, which blocks ultraviolet radiation and lowers the rate of skin cancer. Studies in Nigeria and Tanzania have shown that African albinos tend to get cancer or precancerous skin lesions by age twenty, decreasing their breeding prospects and hence their opportunity to pass on their genes.

Light skin, on the other hand, evolved farther away from the equator because humans had to absorb vitamin D, important for bone development, from the sun through their skin. Higher levels of melanin inhibit absorption of vitamin D, creating problems for darker-skinned people who reside further from the equator. In a 1998 study, 15 percent of African American women in the United States had pelvic bone deformities—and, hence, trouble with childbirth—compared to only 2 percent of European American women. The problem is similar to the rickets suffered by Victorian women whose clothing and cultural habits led to insufficient exposure to the sun. Dark-skinned individuals are also at greater risk of frostbite than light-skinned individuals. Lower levels of melanin, resulting in lighter skin color, evolved as an adaptation to northern latitudes. Nasal size and shape also evolved in response to climatic conditions. People native to cold climates tend to have narrower noses to warm incoming air, and people in dry climates also have narrow noses to moisten incoming air. In addition to genetic adaptation, humans are also capable of *acclimation*, or short-term change, such as sweating when they are hot, and *acclimatization*, longer-term physiological changes in red blood cell production, height, and the increase in lung volume that occurs in response to environmental conditions such as poor nutrition or living at high altitudes.

As our early human ancestors migrated from Africa, they left behind the tropical parasites that are still plaguing modern Africans. Their death rates went down and their populations increased. To support their increasing numbers, they adopted slash-and-burn agriculture and cultivated varieties of wheat and barley in the Middle East that spread through neighboring groups to the whole of Eurasia in only 5,000 years. Then, about 10,000 years ago, fertilization made sedentary agriculture possible, and migration slowed until a new phase was stimulated by the development of seagoing vessels and nomadic pastoralism between 4000 and 3000 B.C. In the long evolutionary relationship of humans and disease, the migration of *Homo sapiens* out of Africa and the development of settled agriculture are two of the most important events. The migration explains why some of our diseases are not only so old, descended with us from our common primate ancestors, but why they are common in humans around the world. And while migration to cooler zones may have reduced the old disease load, settled agriculture allowed humans to stay in one place and have much closer and more frequent contact with each other and with animals, creating the opportunity for transmission of new parasites between humans and their beasts.

More agricultural innovations stimulated another phase of population growth, increasing the crowding in human settlements, creating more opportunities for rapid transmission of parasites from one human to another and between humans and other insect and animal carriers, such as the rats and fleas responsible for the plague. Other human health problems and genetic changes developed in response to settled farming and animal husbandry; one is lactase deficiency, the common allergy to milk that develops in children after four years of age. In groups of European origin, whose ancestors started dairy farming 12,000 years ago, the rate is very low, but it is very high in populations that do not practice dairy farming. Later technological advances—colonization, trade, war, industrialization, and public health and medicine—also caused the human relationship with microbes to change many times over.

Up until several thousand years ago, most of the continent of Africa was covered with dense forests where malarial mosquitoes could not survive. With the advent of horticulture, the malaria mosquito flourished in cleared forests with rain pools and sunlight. As the human population grew, the malarial parasite flourished as well. So as human culture, in the form of agriculture, changed the environment, the environment in turn caused a change in human genetic composition to favor the sickle cell allele. Hemoglobin, a protein in red blood cells, transports oxygen to body tissues. The normal hemoglobin genotype is AA, but the A allele can mutate into other variations, including S. A person with two S alleles has sickle cell anemia, which alters the structure of the red blood cells and impairs oxygen transport. Only about 15 percent of individuals with this genotype survive to adulthood, resulting in 100,000 deaths per year.

Because the mutant S allele is harmful, in most populations it is "bred out" and occurs in very low numbers. However, in African populations with high exposure to malaria, it is found in 5 to 20 percent of all individuals because the blood cells of a person with the AS variant are shaped differently, reducing the harm done by the malaria parasite without resulting in the fatal anemia a person with the SS genotype has. High frequencies of sickle cell are found in sub-Saharan Africa, North Africa, Mediterranean Europe, India, and South Asia, all areas with high levels of malaria. When too many people have the AS type, however, the chance that children with the SS type will be born and suffer from sickle cell anemia grows. These children will not breed, lowering the presence of the S allele in the population as a whole and keeping the system in balance.

Other adaptations to malaria—Hemoglobin C in northwest Africa, G6PD deficiency in the Mediterranean, hemoglobin E in Southeast Asia, and Melanesian ovaloctosis—are similar "scorched earth defenses," protecting carriers with one copy of a mutant allele but killing offspring with two. The spread of these traits through a population is not a problem until the gene becomes so common that children begin inheriting it from both parents. At that point, the death rate of these children acts as a brake against the trait's spread into subsequent generations. In African Americans, the S allele is less common because malaria is no longer endemic in the United States and natural selection has had time to reduce the number of people with the allele. Studies in Britain and the United States have found that fertility is higher among women with the sickle cell trait.

In a similar way, cystic fibrosis results when a child inherits two copies of a gene that in singular form protects its carrier against *Salmonella typhi*, the bacterium causing typhoid fever. With a single copy of the mutant gene, the body produces a protein that hinders the ability of the bacterium to attach to the intestinal lining, although the bacterium can continue to perform its normal activities. Cystic fibrosis is the tragic price paid for protection against typhoid fever, and evolved because prior to the twentieth century, *S. typhi* was ubiquitous in contaminated water and infected almost everyone early in life, killing about 5 percent of all Europeans. These kinds of "costly" adaptations are the way nature maintains a delicate balancing act among microbes and human defenses by affecting human success in reproduction. Crude defenses like these typically originate in simple mutations of only one gene's primary function that emerge from the interaction of a microbe and its human host. First the microbe increases, prompting the selection and spread of a defensive genetic mutation in the group. The disease declines, so the population builds. But when there are more people with the single copy, more children can get one copy of the mutation from both parents and suffer debilitating diseases. As they die, the number of people with the adaptive mutation declines, and the disease increases again. This is one example of what biologist Paul Ewald calls the coevolution of diseases and humans because both the microbe and the human adjust to changes in one another.

While the relationship between the sickle cell allele and malaria is the best-known example of natural selection on a genetic trait, human blood groups, especially ABO, also show the effect of adaptation to disease pressure.

Different blood groups have different antibodies, implying variable resistance to diseases. Variations in ABO blood types result from historical encounters with a wide range of infectious diseases, including smallpox, typhoid, influenza, and bubonic plague. Type A is more susceptible to smallpox, B to infantile diarrhea, and O to bubonic plague.

In nonhuman animals with HIV-type viruses (cows, horses, sheep, and monkeys), the virus and host have coadapted so that the virus is benign, suggesting that these animals have carried the virus for a longer time than humans and that HIV came into existence before humans and chimps reached their divide on the evolutionary tree. Viruses like HIV, herpes, and chicken pox remain latent in humans after initial symptoms disappear, a special talent that makes biologists believe these viruses are very old.[3] Another clue that HIV may have "cohabited" with humans for a very long time is that some humans appear to have partial genetic immunity to the virus. Some prostitutes in Nairobi, Kenya have immune systems that fight off HIV infection as long as they keep having sex. Other Africans also may have some natural immunity to HIV, given the fact that infection levels have stabilized in some countries for no apparent reason but are soaring well beyond the expected ceiling of 30 percent infected in other countries.

A genetic trait discovered in 1994 that gives its carriers some immunity to HIV is found in several Caucasian populations in frequencies high enough to suggest nonrandom spread and selection in response to a specific threat. Scientists theorize that the trait may have arisen as an adaptive response to the bubonic plague. Unlike adaptations to typhoid and malaria, however, having two copies of this gene is even better than having one because people with two copies resist HIV infection entirely while people with one copy can get HIV but its progress is slowed. The mutation is most common in Sweden, where 20 percent of the population carries one or two copies, and its frequency tapers down as you travel south in Europe. Only a small percent of Central Asians carry the mutation, which is absent from the rest of the world. The pattern may reflect differences in the spread of pneumonic plague, transmitted through the air, versus bubonic plague, transmitted through rats and fleas. Europe suffered many waves of plague from the Black Death in 1347 through 1650, when the disease finally began to disappear, possibly as a result of rapid buildup of resistance through this genetic mutation.

✳ ✳ ✳

Paul Ewald calls parasites, including those that cause disease, "evolution's greatest success stories," existing wherever there is life and adapting to every conceivable ecological niche. Four of every five species on earth are parasites when varieties of bacteria, protozoa, fungi, algae, plants and animals that have adopted parasitic survival strategies are included. There were sixty-seven organisms in the dust Darwin gathered from the *Beagle*'s deck, but every pail of seawater used to swab those decks contained 10 billion viruses. Microbes constitute 5 percent of our body weight, multiply luxuriously in our intestines, cover our skin, line our mouths, noses, and other orifices. We are born with our mother's bugs, but the complement inside begins to change immediately after birth as we adjust to our new environment, a process that continues throughout our lives. If we upset the normal balance, diarrhea, vaginitis, bad breath, and body odor result. Bugs in our guts make the vitamins we need for our survival and help us digest our food. Benevolent microbes fend off disease-causing microbes that invade our systems.

Since most bacteria are not dangerous to or even symbiotic with other species, it is likely that they evolved much earlier than any of their insect, plant, or animal hosts. Although we and other hosts are besieged by microbes, most of them do not cause infections. Different kinds of microbes acquired the ability to cause disease as they overcame their hosts' barriers to initial colonization, developed strategies for sharing their nutrients, avoided their hosts' defense systems, replicated, and found a way to infect new hosts. Mechanisms for colonization and symbiosis, or the ability to live off their hosts, are similar in all pathogens, whether they colonize plant or animal hosts. Benign microbe strains also acquire the set of genes for symbiosis and the set that allows them to avoid host defenses before they can acquire the set of genes necessary to become pathogenic. After this genetic set evolves, deadly microbes can pass it on as a complete trait to benign microbes, and if they are favored by natural selection, the microbes with the deadly DNA survive. This ability considerably speeds up the process of benign microbes becoming deadly killers and explains how some diseases spread so quickly in our bodies.

The defense and survival systems of some pathogens are so powerful that they can totally alter the host species' behavior to ensure their own reproductive success. For example, a strain of bacteria known as *Wolbachia* makes it impossible for uninfected hosts to breed by producing a toxin that alters the male's sperm and an antidote that restores sperm to viability if the female is infected. The bacterium's survival strategy is so effective that it has caused speciation at least once by separating uninfected and infected wasps. Biologists are looking at how this capacity could be used to attack widespread diseases like malaria, elephantitis, and river blindness, in which the bacterium plays an important role in causing the inflammation that leads to blindness. The bacteria infects up to 76 percent of all nonvertebrates, including shrimp, spiders, and all types of insects.

Using a "family tree" approach, genetic analyses feasible only in the last ten years have demonstrated the relative antiquity of many human pathogens. By comparing viral and bacterial family trees with the geographic distributions of a disease, researchers can infer the age and routes of a disease's geographic spread. For example, *Trypanosoma brucei* causes sleeping sickness, which still kills about 300,000 Africans each year, while its cousin, *Trypanosoma cruzi*, causes Chagas' disease, Darwin's affliction, which infects 20 million people around the world. In 2001 British researchers showed that the two trypanosomes branched from a common ancestor 100 million years ago when Africa, South America, and Australia were joined in one continent called Gondwana. Africa split from the main continent first, so that modern trypanosomes have an African group and an "all-other" group similar to the two main human genetic groups in the world. Through coevolution, some humans now carry an "anti-tryp" factor in their blood that prevents the disease, but not all human groups have evolved this antidote. The bacterium that causes stomach ulcers, *Helicobacter pylori*, was identified in 1982, and its genetic family tree has a European branch and an East Asian branch. This split occurred when the first African migrants, who were carrying the disease, reached the Middle East and from there set out in opposite directions. These differences in any bacteria's genetic lineages are so useful they have prompted biologists to start reconstructing early human migrations using bacteria.

With the capability for tracing genetic family trees, scientists now know that many human diseases are very old, dating from before humans developed settled agriculture. Recent analyses show that some diseases we thought originated from domesticated animals actually originated in humans who passed them to their beasts. The closest relatives of human tapeworms, for example, are not in cows or pigs, but in East African antelopes, lions, and hyenas. The American team examining this disease thinks that "as hominids made the shift from herbivory to carnivory, they were exposed to these tapeworms" because they scavenged the carcasses of animal predators. The tapeworm coevolved with its human host and was transferred to cows and pigs several hundred thousand years later.

Genetic typing has determined that other diseases are also very old. Dysentery, unknown in any other species, is caused by bacteria that burrow into human intestinal walls. Australian biologists have found that the bacteria that causes it, *Shigella*, evolved from more two harmless *E. coli* strains, both of which existed before humans separated from chimps. Researchers suspect that anthrax and tuberculosis also may be much older than formerly believed. Hepatitis C, only identified in 1989, infects 170 million people and is related to viruses in the Flaviviridae family, which also includes dengue and yellow fevers. It is much older than HIV because it is much more diverse, but like HIV, it did not flare until fifty to eighty years ago. The benign Hepatitis G virus, discovered in 1995, infects 5 to 15 percent of the world's population. Unlike its distant cousin C, many versions of G have been found in primates. Its genetic tree has two main divisions, Old World and New World, so the virus probably separated into two species when its human hosts separated. In 1998 South American researchers sequencing the genes of various types of *Falciparium* malaria found that they are descended from a common ancestor that is 500,000 years old.

Although most of our disease-causing parasites are very old, some, like *Yersis pestis*, the cause of the bubonic plague, are not. *Y. pestis* evolved from a bacterium shed in rodent feces sometime in the last 2,000 years. Syphilis, while related to a much older disease, yaws, has a slightly different genetic sequence and probably evolved more recently. Scientists began scanning samples from around the world in 1998. When available, the results will show us when this sexually transmitted disease (STD) evolved. HIV, like syphilis, appears to be an old disease that only recently evolved into a pathogen. If the age of human STDs can be estimated, it may provide a clue about their purpose in human evolution.

All pathogens evolve sophisticated survival strategies so they will not be killed by their host cells and to get themselves passed on to new hosts. Ewald likens STDs to "criminals living in a town that is heavily patrolled by police." Syphilis is like a thief that sands off his fingerprints, stripping off external molecules to make itself unrecognizable. HIV disguises itself as a police officer by dressing in the immune cell's own membrane. Gonorrhea bacteria change their disguises, wearing different external molecules daily, and use the reproductive tract as a hideout. They trash it in the process, but not enough to cause an immune response. Herpes simplex hides out in the nervous system, while human papillomaviruses "are the organized criminals. They take over the cells of the cervix, making them work for the new boss," forcing them to divide more rapidly than is good for the body, and fooling the immune system by using the body's own cells. If each of these pathogens seems to be exhibiting extraordinarily sophisticated behavior, consider *Wolbachia*, which manipulates its host so well that that it forces it to form new species. All of these behaviors have developed through years of adaptation to the host species.

While microbes are essential to our survival, our relationship with them is competitive. Parasites must consume their host to survive, forcing their host to defend itself. These twin imperatives create a "fierce co-evolutionary struggle" according to biologist Carl Zimmer. As we evolve, microbes make changes, and vice versa. Darwin discovered the principle of coevolution by observing the interaction of plants and their insect pollinators, which, "either simultaneously or one after the other, modified and adapted in the most perfect manner to each other, by continued preservation of individuals presenting mutual and slightly favorable deviations of structure." Later scientists discovered that coevolution is even more widespread than Darwin realized. Only 10 percent of all plants can spread their pollen by wind or water. The rest depend on insects or animals for fertilization. Many species of plants depend on the colonies of fungus around their roots to extract nutrients from the soil, which in turn consume about 15 percent of the plants' nutrients. Some fungi also kill insect and parasite enemies and help plants resist droughts and other disasters. In the same way, human digestion and other functions are aided by a multitude of "friendly" parasites, and we must be careful not to upset our relationship with them. Antibiotics kill friendly flora in human stomachs that must be replenished; douching kills friendly parasites in human vaginas. The cream and gel microbicides developed for use by women to protect themselves from HIV transmission also kill friendly microbes necessary to the vagina's balanced ecology.

More serious in the fight against the epidemic is the ability of HIV to mutate and evolve in its coevolution with its human host, evading the drugs taken to suppress it and hindering the development of an effective vaccine. HIV mutates within the body of an infected individual, developing resistant strains as the body's immune system fights back. Each time the immune system succeeds, the virus evolves again, and "without an HIV test," says Zimmer, "infected people have no way of knowing that a coevolutionary struggle is raging under their own skin." HIV drugs must be updated constantly and used in changing combinations to defeat the virus's strategy, but "the virus's mutational overdrive is already threatening to make them useless."

✳ ✳ ✳

Some of the most surprising findings of evolutionary research over the past 100 years concern the interrelationship of sex and disease, without which human evolution would not have been possible. The presence of disease also shapes the biological mechanisms of sex and reproduction in many members of the animal kingdom and their mating behaviors, the social and individual acts that make the biological process possible. Disease is the engine of diversity in all plant and animal populations, and through that diversity, it makes them healthier in three ways. The obvious one is to kill off individuals with "bad" genes, who are weaker and more susceptible to diseases, before they have a chance to mate. Death eventually happens to us all, but disease determines how much time between puberty and old age we get to pass on our genes. Recall the example of albinos in Africa, most of whom die before they have the opportunity to reproduce. People with disabilities in developing countries also die faster, while modern medicine helps many people in developed countries overcome the constraints of genetic defects and disabilities and mate.

The second way disease interacts with reproduction is to reduce the likelihood that individuals with less advantageous genes will mate. Because of the early presence of disease in their lives or that of their families, some individuals are smaller and less robust than others. In the animal world, and to some degree in the human world, they lose out to larger, more robust individuals. The mating contests like those described in *The Origin of the Species* determine which males get to mate and pass on their genes. In many animal groups, an alpha male has command of an entire herd of females and mates exclusively with them until a stronger male successfully challenges his monopoly.

The third way disease impacts sex and mating is much less obvious. Darwin figured out the basics, but it took another hundred or so years for biologists to paint in the details. The first thing disease does is to encourage *sexual*, as opposed to *asexual*, reproduction, and through that to encourage the genetic mixing that provides the opportunity for healthful innovation in animal species. Sex is an evolutionary adaptation in all humans, in most mammals, and in some members of the plant kingdom. Few asexual animals are known even though, in many ways, asexual reproduction seems more efficient because everyone can do it and no one has to use any energy to fight or compete for attention. In the whiptail lizard, one female mimics male lizard behavior and mounts another, bites her neck, and wraps around her midsection, causing the second to ovulate. The egg, without fertilization by sperm, starts to divide and grow into embryos. The "female" then mounts the "male" so she too can reproduce, and both bear female clones of themselves. Yet there are many more sexual animals than asexual ones, said Darwin. "Peacocks show no sign of evolving away their tails; new generations of redback spider males are throwing themselves into the jaws of death just as their fathers did."

Since Darwin's time, biologists have found that the answer to this biological paradox lies in disease. Sex fights off parasites because the combination of genes from a male and a female generates variation in offspring so that any population that practices sexual reproduction has a better chance of surviving. Cloning produces no variation, so if a fatal parasite invades a whiptail lizard population and no individual has immunity through a mutation, all the whiptail lizards die. Parasites and populations coevolve, running in cycles of boom and crash. When parasites are successful, they eventually kill off most of their hosts and die off as well. Their host population begins its boom cycle, and the "deadly merry-go-round" circles again, says Zimmer. Since only the host with immunity has survived, it thrives until a new parasite comes along. Sexual activity gradually allows a thorough mixing of genes. When parasites attack, they can no longer "force them into boom-and-bust cycles as dramatic as the ones suffered by their clonal cousins." Sexual reproduction works so well, it has "come in to existence dozens of times, in many separate lineages of animals, plants, red algae, and other eukaryotes," Zimmer says.

The mechanics of fertilization have evolved a similar form in many species. A big immobile egg and a lot of small, fast-swimming sperm increase the probability that at least one sperm will reach its target and fertilization will occur. But while the mechanics of fertilization work very efficiently, when pregnancy occurs there is another bottleneck. One male can fertilize many females, but they still have to go through a period of pregnancy and nurse the offspring that are born, making fewer females available for breeding at any one time. Sexual selection breaks this bottleneck because it determines which males get to mate. Males may battle over females and the victor takes the spoils, but most mating contests are much more subtle. "The sight of a feather in a peacock's tail...makes me sick!" Darwin exclaimed, frustrated by his inability to deduce why the male bird has tail feathers so heavy they burden his flight. After several years observing leks, or groups of peacocks during mating season, he had his answer. As they spread out their tails, the males call to the females, who are drawn to the shivering display of feathers. The male with the biggest, most symmetrical tail wins, making female choice a critical force in evolution. Peahens will cluster around the male peacock with the largest, most elaborate, most symmetrical tail, and males with fewer than 130 "eyes" on their tails probably will not mate. Hens like roosters with the biggest combs, female swordfish prefer bigger swords, and female crickets like males with complicated calls.

For more than hundred years after Darwin published his findings, geneticists remained puzzled. Why does the peahen "like" the bigger tail? What makes it sexy enough to be reproduced even though it was a potential threat to survival? Displays like these also make a demand on the male's energy, and natural selection puts a ceiling on their elaboration. A male peacock with a tail that is too large cannot fly from a pursuing fox. The answer, once again, lies in resistance to disease. A peahen with fewest parasites will have a better chance of reproducing successfully and passing on her genes if she picks the male with fewest parasites. While the peahen "cannot send her suitor's genes to a laboratory for analysis," Zimmer says, she can look at his tail; "to sing loudly or grow bright feathers, a male can't be too weakened by his fight with parasites." A rooster with a large comb has produced a lot of testosterone to grow it, lowering his immunity and putting himself at risk. If he can do that and still be strong, his immune system must be very strong. Symmetry is also a good sign that the peacock's mother was strong enough to fight off stresses in the womb that might leave marks on her young while they were still in the embryonic stage. Humans, male and female alike, think that humans with more symmetrical facial features are more "beautiful" and also prefer taller individuals over short ones, both signs of strong immune systems.

Disease affects the choices of mating individuals through clear physical clues that help potential mates make "healthy" choices, mating with individuals that are least burdened by pathogens. Even "promiscuity"—mating with many partners—is a behavior that acts to reduce pathogens and increase evolutionary fitness of the population overall. The ringer, of course, is when an STD is present and quickly spreads to a much wider group because of promiscuity, the overall adaptive level of the group is reversed. Scientists, long aware that promiscuity is the norm in the animal world, recently found that it is prevalent in birds as well. Naturalists believed that 90 percent of bird species were monogamous. Since it takes two birds to raise chicks successfully, scientists assumed they were committed pairs. But genetic testing on chicks of some species shows an illegitimacy rate of up to 55 percent. Females who mate with males that are less than top shelf are more likely to cheat, offsetting the genetic shortcomings of their partner by mating with more desirable males that come visiting, while maintaining their helpmate to raise the chicks when they are born. This ensures that genes for strong immune systems are more widely dispersed in the population because successful males still get to mate with a broad group of females while preserving the appearance of monogamy. Promiscuity slows the rapid narrowing of the genetic base of a group, so that if an epidemic strikes, at least some individuals will have immunity to it and survive.

In the world of chimps, females find their mates outside of the group where they were born and spend 70 percent of their lives away from their home groups, but never bond with females in their mate's group. "As a result, male chimps have all the power," Zimmer says, because they form alliances for hunting and food gathering. Males are very violent toward the females and murder babies sired by other males. In this setting, promiscuity makes sense to protect the young. When a female chimp is ready, she mates with as many males as possible, having sex on average 138 times with 13 different males for every baby conceived. As a result, the males are unable to determine which one is the father and are less likely to kill the baby. Widespread mating also increases networking and group solidarity. Primary sexual characteristics in some animals are directly related to the number of sperm they must produce to ensure they win in a multimate lottery. Among primate species, average testicle size is directly proportional to the average number of partners the females mate with. "The more intense the competition, the more sperm a male primate produces," says Zimmer.

In another species of primate, the bonobo (more closely related to humans than the chimp), females are dominant and suffer very little violence from the males. No babies are threatened with infanticide because the females form strong bonds among themselves. In this society, sex is not just for reproduction and is not used to protect babies. It is used to diffuse tensions and make alliances in the group. Female bonobos are in heat 50 percent of the time, while chimps are sexually accessible only 5 percent of the time. Bonobos have sex when they discover new food sources, Zimmer says, instead of fighting like chimps, and "if a male has a fit of jealousy and chases another male away from a female bonobo, the two males may later reunite for some scrotal rubbing." Males and females both have sex with same sex partners, deescalating competition. They live in a much richer environment than chimps, so there is no conflict between groups: "when two groups of bonobos meet up, they have sex rather than fight."

Many human sexual habits are evolutionary adaptations that have clear explanations in the world of biology. While we may prefer to think of the human species and ourselves as monogamous, in humans, as in birds, appearances are deceiving. Humans, like birds, are a promiscuous species, or, as Cornell anthropologist Meredith Small prefers to put it, a "*mildly* polygynous species, one that has evolved from a *highly* polygynous species."[4] In polygynous mating systems, males have many mates. Polygyny is a special case of the more familiar term "polygamy," describing mating systems in which both males and females have more than one partner. Small believes that humans are on their way to monogamy but have not quite finished their evolutionary transformation from polygamy. Humans still retain some of the genetic coding for the social behavior of their ancestors. Small, who studies the sexual behavior of primates, says that the size difference between human males and females is a dead giveaway. As Darwin suggested a long time ago after noting that males outsize females in many species, natural selection favors bigger males in mating systems where males compete for females. In the 14 percent of primate species that favor monogamy and live in pairs, males and females are much closer in body size. Baboon males, on the other hand, are two times the size of females because the winner of the sexual competition gets to mate with all the females (at least for a while) and pass his genes down to more baboons in the next generation.

Human females are, on average, 80 percent of the size of human males, indicating that while monogamy may be a cultural ideal for some of us, we have not quite turned it into a reality. In fact, only 16 percent of human societies even claim to be monogamous; the other 84 percent actually call themselves polygamous. This, however, is somewhat misleading, as anthropologists who have spent untold numbers of hours classifying marriage systems know. What people say they do and what they actually do are two very different things. In most polygamous societies, only the richest males, about 10 percent, can actually afford more than one wife at a time. The rest content themselves with "serial monogamy," marrying (or mating with) one person at a time but more than one partner in a lifetime.

Men and women all over the world are adulterous; in 73 percent of cultures worldwide married men and women report that they have had other partners while married. In the 1970s women began catching up with men, although in most cultures more men take on new partners than women. In every society men report that they want four times as many sex partners as women do, have more sexual fantasies, and let less time elapse before seeking sex with a new partner. Men are also more willing to have sex with a total stranger. Small also argues that we are like our primate relatives in several other respects. The pleasure of sexuality pushes us toward mating, but Small argues that we humans "tend to exaggerate our sexuality at this point in our evolution," so that "sexuality defines so much of our culture and our lives."

The human male has a much larger penis than his closest relatives, chimps (including bonobos) and gorillas, but relatively small testicles, larger than gorillas but much smaller than chimps. While we know testicle size is correlated with sperm production, no one has quite figured out why the human penis is so large. It grows exponentially during puberty, when male-male competition for females begins. Small suggests that, like the peacock's tail display, the human penis may be large to attract females or that it evolved to frighten away other males. It may have evolved to enhance male or female sexual pleasure, but this idea has not been scientifically evaluated. The evolutionary cause for the large human penis can only be guessed. Perhaps it coevolved, like the tongues of Madagascar moths and the necks of the orchids they fertilize that Darwin studied, gaining length as the vagina gained depth.

After completing a lengthy study of the sex lives of orchids, Darwin realized their shapes "were not for beauty's sake, but elaborate devices for luring insects into their sex lives."

In many species, it helps to have both mates around to raise the offspring, but in humans as in chimps, females bear much of the load. Males are often absent, and they do not provide much support in foraging, feeding, or discipline. While the relatively small contribution of men to the family in many developing countries is often a function of poverty, too much work, or labor migration, there may be some genetic or biological component as well because it is also found among men in developed countries. Females of all species, including humans, bear the responsibilities of pregnancy and nursing, and they look for males who will support and nurture their offspring. Human females are universally attracted to older, more stable men who can support them while they are pregnant and vulnerable. Men, on the other hand, prefer younger women and are sexually attracted to a body type with proportions that suggest high fertility. Small reports that it is more stressful for a man to think of his partner having sex with someone else than becoming emotionally attached to another person, while a woman is more stressed by the thought that her man will abandon her than by the idea that he might have had a one-night stand. The infanticide of unrelated offspring seen in other species is found in humans too. A child is 40 to 100 times more likely to be killed by a stepparent than by a biological parent, and being a stepchild is the strongest risk factor for child abuse.

Human mating may be somewhat universal in its patterns, but human marriage systems vary a great deal in the importance they give to the male-female bond and in the living arrangements of men and women. Where economic conditions allow and modernization encourages, men and women who marry generally try to establish their own households as soon as possible. In African societies, the male-female marriage bond is especially weak, and Australian anthropologist Caldwell says, "virtue is related more to success in reproduction than to limiting profligacy." Women and men remain more closely tied to their own families than to their marriage partners, a holdover from unstable economic and social systems. The pattern of high fertility makes sense, too, in the context of African history, where death from disease and famine always has been high and dislocation from any number of sources—slavery, colonialism, forced labor, soldiery—has been more common than peaceful social life. In addition, African farming systems are labor intensive, which encourages women to have more children. With no other social security systems in place, older members of families must rely on their children to support them in their old age. High fertility, under these circumstances, is closely related to the need for social stability. The human inclination to mate with more than one partner, coupled with weak partner bonds, high social instability, and economic systems that encourage high fertility, makes it especially easy for any STD to spread quickly. In addition, the low productivity of subsistence agriculture and lack of alternative employment in Africa's rural areas encourages men and women to migrate to urban areas to find work to support their families. In the process, they are not only freed from the social constraints implicit in traditional village life, but suffer the alienation and loneliness that encourage them to seek other bonds. All of these conditions coincide to hasten frequent multiple partner sex, and set the stage for rampant STD epidemics.

✕ ✕ ✕

In their competition with humans, "microbes have the advantage. There are a lot more of them than us. Their generation time is minutes instead of years. They evolve rapidly. And, of course, we aid and abet them in many ways—by travel, commerce in foodstuffs, transportation of animals, and our abuse and overuse of antibiotics. We're playing right into their hands,"[5] says veteran epidemic observer Rick Weiss. They are so powerful that Joshua Lederberg, president emeritus of the Rockefeller University in New York, wonders why humans managed to survive at all. (Microbes are not our only predators, but they are our most fearsome.) Humans have responded through cultural, scientific, behavioral, social, economic, and political means, but microbes usually come out the winners. Nothing is stagnant in the world of bugs, so our relationship to them will always be coevolutionary. By better understanding the impact of our actions on the intimate world of disease-causing agents and their vectors, our coevolution will result in continued adaptive success for both parties.

In 1942 microbiologist René Dubos, who ushered in the age of antibiotics, warned that "it is a dangerous error to believe that disease and suffering can be wiped out altogether by raising still further the standards of living, increasing our mastery of the environment, and developing new therapeutic procedures. The less pleasant reality is that, since the world is ever changing, each period and each type of civilization will continue to have its burden of diseases created by unavoidable failure of biological and social adaptation to counter new threats." Dubos' caution was overrun by clamoring optimism for medical miracles at the end of World War II, stimulated by his discoveries. Lederburg says that the human race has had many "close calls," including the flu epidemic of 1918 and the Black Death, but that "with rare exceptions, our microbial adversaries have had a shared interest in our survival." If we die, they do too; if they kill us all, they will have no more hosts and will become extinct. Lederberg reasoned that "the pathogenic species will find it to their advantage to evolve in a way that reduces their virulence." Short-term flare-ups come with new mutants that do not follow established rules.

Until recently, most microbiologists assumed that bugs "played fair." Then Paul Ewald hypothesized that this assumption applied only to microbes passed from person to person because an infected individual must still be able to make contact with others. Waterborne infections and infections transmitted by insects can be much more lethal because they do not have to keep their host alive very long. Cholera, for example, is much more deadly in areas where water and sewer systems are not very clean because an infected person can pass the bacteria on quickly. In these circumstances, the bug has no need to keep a carrier alive for long. Where sanitation systems are cleaner, a less virulent strain of cholera predominates because it has to keep the person alive longer before it is transmitted.

Different strains of a disease microbe with different levels of virulence live side by side in groups and individuals, where they compete for dominance. Even a common bacteria like *E. coli* can include a wide array of variants, mixes, or combinations, as HIV does. To Ewald, the competition of microbes with a human's immune system is a miniature evolutionary struggle. Microbes enter a new environment, just as people do, testing the multiple mutations produced in their rapid breeding cycles. When the body responds with defenses, the microbe population is modified; less well-adapted mutations die out and more successful ones, for example, those that are resistant to an antibiotic, continue to survive. If the adaptive process is successful, the bug population increases. Ewald believes that HIV has existed in humans for decades, if not hundreds or millions of years, and that socioeconomic upheaval in the 1960s and 1970s encouraged the emergence of more virulent strains. In Africa and in the world as a whole, rapid spread of STDs coincided with rapid population growth and urbanization. The dense host populations of cities are good news for any pathogen because the number of contacts between infected people and uninfected or susceptible people increases. Rates of HIV and other STDs are higher in urban than in rural populations because of the breakdown in social inhibitions and traditional institutions in cities, increased opportunity for men to make anonymous visits to sex workers there, and the opportunity for sexually active people to make contact with many more potential mates.

Unlike other microbes that get themselves passed on by making their host sneeze or scratch, a frequent act, STDs rely on sexual transmission, a less frequent act. STDs must persist in their human hosts for a relatively long time while waiting to be transmitted to new hosts. As far as STDs are concerned, the diseases they cause while they wait are only what Ewald calls "the cost of doing business." STD survival strategies are sound from their viewpoint. While costly to their host, Ewald points out that "the cost of no sex is higher" from an evolutionary perspective. To pass on your genes, it is vastly more important to have sex than avoid it because you are afraid of getting an STD or of passing one on; that is, if you even know you have one. A more virulent HIV strain predominates in an individual carrying one or more strains if he or she has many sex partners and can frequently transmit it. If the infected person has no sex partners or has sex less frequently, the less virulent strains predominate because the virus must be able to survive long enough to be passed on.

At the individual level, increased sexual activity encourages takeover by the more virulent strain. At the population level, when there is less sexual activity, virulence declines overall. Bacterial STDs follow this pattern, as do papillomaviruses, which are milder in women with fewer than five sexual partners, increase in virulence in women with six to ten partners, and are three times more lethal in women who have had more than ten lifetime partners. During the war in Yugoslavia, in a population that previously had the least virulent strains of papillomavirus, wartime rapes caused the lethal types to become three times more prevalent. Herpes also becomes worse with increases in general stress and sexual activity. HIV may be becoming less virulent with changes in sexual behavior in Africa. However, the Nairobi prostitutes who are genetically immune to HIV are an exception. When they stop having sex or have it less frequently, they are more likely to become HIV positive. Perhaps the children born with the infection, who become HIV negative when their own antibodies refuse to establish a coevolutionary relationship with the microbe, are being genetically selected over the long term for their high resistance. Perhaps the Nairobi prostitutes are the offspring of such relationships a long time ago. Continentwide, 9 percent of all Africans are HIV positive. This either means that the sexual behavior of 91 percent is such that they have not contracted HIV, or that there is a considerable level of natural immunity. These levels vary quite a bit in different countries, but even in the most infected countries, sizable segments of the population remain uninfected.

STDs, enormously clever and destructive microbes, have existed at relatively high levels in human beings since at least the 1500s, and have infected ever more human beings over the last forty years since the introduction of birth control methods that do not require a condom or other barriers to transmission. The prevalence of all types of STDs is increasing worldwide with increased sexual behavior. Ewald thinks that as "people start having sex with more people or with less protection, venereal pathogens will not only spread but evolve to become more harmful." The most effective prevention method is clinical detection and treatment. Public education campaigns are not informative enough to inspire caution. Most people are still badly informed about the gravity of STDs and their contribution to cancer, paralysis, infertility, congenital birth defects, arthritis, Alzheimer's disease, and heart disease.

STDs seem to controvert the very purpose defined by Darwin for individuals of any species to improve fitness and transmission of their genes. Since STDs reduce fertility and sexual pleasure, they hinder an infected person's ability to reproduce. Infection also leads to fatal and disabling conditions in offspring, reducing the reproductive potential of parents and children both. Young people are more likely to contract HIV and other STDs, die young, and have fewer children. Under these circumstances, from an evolutionary point of view it makes sense for one or both infected partners to avoid sex. Avoidance is possible with some STDs, but most have long latency periods and few symptoms in their early stages. Someone with syphilis, HIV, or many other STDs can have many contacts before the infection becomes visible or known to the person who carries it.

It is tempting to think that if there is a long-term evolutionary benefit of STDs to the human species, it is to lower population density through deaths and to slow population growth by reducing fertility. It is, indeed, a cruel check on population growth, but as Darwin pointed out, perhaps STDs are like the ceiling on the growth of peacocks' tails. Male peacocks with excessive testosterone levels eventually end up with too many tail feathers and are eaten by predators when they can no longer take rapid flight from the ground. If that were not the case, eventually one male would dominate the lek and breed with all the females, reducing the amount of genetic diversity and, in the long run, resistance to disease. Perhaps the evolutionary function of STDs is to reduce the reproductive potential of individuals in human populations with high hormone levels whose genes might otherwise dominate the group.

While we wait for an HIV vaccine or a cure for AIDS, HIV is gaining vital time to build up a huge reservoir of infections and to create resistant strains with higher virulence. A vaccine or a cure is likely to be a long time in coming. Vaccines rely on the immune system, but STDs have evolved sophisticated ways to avoid destruction by immune system responses. Hepatitis B, for one, and HIV, for another, stay ahead in the race with the immune system by mutating so that even "if the vaccine primes the immune system to combat one form of the virus, the door is left open for another," Ewald says. The outcomes of protection through vaccination will become obvious only on very long time scales. So far our track record in containing viruses is not very impressive. We still have no cure for the common cold, herpes, or any other disease caused by viruses, and they have been around a whole lot longer than HIV/AIDS.

By increasing our efforts to inform people about the destructiveness of these infections and encouraging them to practice safe sex with a condom, we have an opportunity to apply the principles of coevolution. Safe sex can diminish the virulence of these pathogens and slow their transmission rate, and treatment reduces virulence, slows transmission, and averts some of the longer-term damage to bodily systems experienced by people living with HIV/AIDS. Fortunately, it appears that if young people are informed, they are able to change their sexual behavior, perhaps because they are modifying it before it becomes firmly established. The hypersexuality being encouraged by advertisers and drug manufacturers works against this, however. While humans are genetically programmed to want sex, the level considered necessary is determined by beliefs about what is "normal" and "healthy." We might want to think about the long-term effects on our health of advertisers who promote products with sex and the pervasiveness of sexuality and pornography in modern societies. Better yet, we may have to confront our age-old taboos around frank discussion of sexuality with teens if we hope to help them avoid bearing the burdens imposed by these diseases. Either way, it helps to know that norms are human artifacts, not God-given rules.

❋ ❋ ❋

In 1970 Columbia University anthropologist Alexander Alland realized that the social change caused by our interaction with disease may be as important to evolution as their affect on rates of birth, death, and illness. Our response to disease, Alland wrote, forms a buffer between humans and ever-changing environments and is an expression of human adaptation to environmental pressures. Behavioral changes that are occurring in social, economic, and political systems in Africa and the world in response to HIV/AIDS are examples of these kinds of buffering adaptations. Wider availability of HIV prevention programs, new approaches to treatment, adoption of orphans, and innovative community care programs for AIDS patients and their children are just a few examples. Rising global political discontent in many countries with elites who fail to negotiate broader responses is another.

In 2002, a group of African health program administrators I worked with listed more than fifty positive examples of fundamental social change in Africa and in the international political arena prompted by the HIV/AIDS epidemic. Their examples included openness about sexuality between parents and children, increased maturity and leadership by teenagers, and increased willingness of people from all walks of life to work together in community groups like the ones that were organized by Molly, Robina and Pauline to fight the disease, organize care, and increase social productivity. Programs in Uganda and many other countries show that humans can radically change the way they deal with sexuality without becoming the promiscuous monsters predicted by Victorian morality. In fact, as people become more open about sexuality, sexual activity among teenagers and adults diminishes.

When one-fifth, one-quarter, or one-third of a human population is wiped out in relatively short order—as is occurring now with HIV/AIDS in some countries—many things have got to change. A society's interest groups are brought into conflict as human beings die on a large scale, and economic structures, as Alland and other social scientists have noted, are often those in deepest conflict with health structures. The battle of human rights groups against U.S.-led World Trade Organization policies that protect the high profits of pharmaceutical companies while denying many people with AIDS low-cost generic drugs that could prolong their lives is but one example.

In response to the AIDS epidemic, education systems are being modernized rapidly in Africa, and many more countries now provide free universal primary education, education about AIDS and sexuality, and wide access to condoms. African societies are evolving positively with changes that ensure that future generations are better educated, that orphans are socialized, and that young people learn how to negotiate themselves safely through the health and social challenges of adolescence in the time of AIDS. Businesses are now providing much more comprehensive healthcare for their employees. Farmers in many countries have adapted by cultivating communal fields, which reduces labor requirements and increases yields. The wide-ranging responses of heavily infected societies may place them at an advantage in their competition with developed countries that have stagnated in their actions and attitudes toward sexuality.

Africans are becoming more aware of the role of poverty in illness because of the HIV/AIDS epidemic and recognize how global economic and trading systems perpetuate their poverty, leading to increased malnutrition, susceptibility to disease, and the spread of HIV/AIDS. They are demanding debt forgiveness and fair trade rules so they can begin to catch up financially and make the investment in social systems needed to respond to the epidemic.

And they are demanding the medical care that will help them get through the epidemic with most of their resources intact. Thus the epidemic is promoting a fundamental change in the relationship of African countries to the rest of the world and a new awareness in developed countries of how our lifestyles consume resources poor people in other countries desperately need to survive.

HIV/AIDS illness and deaths on an unprecedented scale are calling forth social responses on an equally unprecedented scale, as illness and death did during the long period when the bubonic plague threatened European countries. In cities and towns, humans drew together to control that plague and established committees to manage their responses. After a brief phase of denial about AIDS, the communities of Little Africa organized themselves to go on. As Molly, Robina, Pauline, and the chiefs are demonstrating, African women and men in every country, often provoked to action by the desperation of surviving orphans, have picked themselves up to care for their ill and dying and provide for their children. To do so, they are calling on deep reserves of strength and their own creative imaginations to find resources, because little has flowed down to them to help. There is a tipping point, however, at which human social systems, no matter how plucky the surviving members are, collapse. Communities that are already deeply poor, living on the margins of subsistence, simply do not have far to fall.

In Africa, the period of denial has passed, but the anger refuses to go away. Africans are very much aware that they are now the victims of genocide by neglect in a world that refuses to share. The rest of the world responded for a short time to the quick starvation produced by African famines, but stood by while the long, slow starvation that is a way of life in many countries opened the door to HIV/AIDS. We stood by and watched the Rwandan massacres occur. In an epidemic, as we have seen, failure to respond is a response.

CHAPTER EIGHT

Evolution and Epidemic Management

Molly looked up from the paper. "My father used to tell us that the Greeks thought their Gods came to Africa once a year on vacation. While they were here, they feasted for twelve days with the 'blameless Ethiopians,' who had gold, elephants, and ebony. Homer said the men down here were the tallest, best-looking and longest-lived in the world."[1] "They obviously hadn't visited Rakai," Robina countered. "Hey," Pauline laughed. "Nobody heard of Rakai until we hit the front page of the *New York Times* as the birthplace of AIDS!"

Save the Children's social welfare officer had brought a copy of the *Times* article on AIDS in Uganda to the women when he came down with their funding contract the week before. Molly looked down at the paper and continued to read. " 'Before Julius Keeya Kintu's father died of AIDS five years ago, he taught his son how to grow coffee, squash and cassava, whose root is Uganda's staple food.' " "Since when did cassava become our staple food?" Pauline interrupted. "Shhh, Pauline. Let Molly go on," Robina chided.

" 'Together they patched up the family's brick-and-thatch hut. Then, a few months ago, Julius's mother, sick with AIDS and unable to care for herself, left her children and traveled to her mother's home to die. Now thirteen, Julius had become the head of the family, the oldest boy of the seven children left to survive on their own on the two hilly acres that yield their scant livelihood.' " Molly looked away. "Is that one of your mini-families, Molly?" Robina asked. "I visit them every few days," Molly replied. "They're in pretty bad shape. I don't think his father taught Julius how to have the strength to go on or to be farmer enough to take care of six other kids. Here, Pauline, why don't you finish reading this?"

Pauline took the paper from Molly and put on her glasses. " 'My father taught me how to plan and my mother, she taught me discipline,' said Julius, a thin wiry boy, his voice low and serious. 'When I am older I want to be a doctor. I see so many people who are sick and they die before they even get to the hospital.' " "He never told me that!" Molly said. "I'm sure he never told you a lot of things, Molly. Let me finish. 'AIDS deaths touch every Ugandan family, mostly the young adults and breadwinners or very young children, and relief workers say fear and emotional exhaustion are overwhelming. The average life span after one is infected with H.I.V. is five years. Hospitals are overcrowded and there is a large market in herbal medicines and in some cases witchcraft to treat disease. Drugs like AZT are not available; infected Ugandans have access only to antibiotics, aspirin, and cortisone cream for skin rashes.' "

"Where'd she see anybody who even had that?" Robina grumbled. "Come on, Pauline, get to the stuff about us." Pauline squinted, running her finger down the text. "Here we are!" she exclaimed. And then she frowned. "At least you, Molly. 'Miss Ssentongo has watched the sickness of parents drive children to suicide, and teenagers numbly cleaning adults who can no longer control their bodies. Her conversations are mostly about AIDS and sexual behavior. Depression shadows her work.' " She stopped and shook her head. "Damn, I don't see anything about the rest of us. Wait a minute. Here's those old folks in Lyantonde. 'The Kabogozas have had to care for eighteen boys and girls, all the offspring of their deceased children. Kabogoza is raising twelve young grand-children. In Rakai, which is home to 380,000 Ugandans, there are approxi-mately 60,000 orphans.' " "What about our project?" Robina demanded.

"Ah, Robina," Pauline said. "Nobody wants to hear about that. All they want to do is shed a little tear over our dead bodies, wring their hands over our horrible fate, and say a little prayer for our miserable black souls. The Greeks may have believed that God lived in Africa, but everyone else seems to have forgotten."

"We can't sit around a wait for them to remember," Robina said. "We have to do what we can. I just hope we can keep some of these children alive and get them into school so they don't become thieves, degenerates, and incorri-gible renegades. I have enough rebels on my hands. And," she paused, fin-gering the condom model on her desk, "we have to teach them how to protect themselves. I only hope it works."

"I'm hoping for a vaccine," Molly muttered. "I'm not sure anybody can really change the way they play sex."

"I'm hoping for a miracle," Pauline sighed, taking off her glasses. She touched one of the spots on her face. "I'm going to need one soon."

"I'm hoping that you two decide to get to work!" Robina laughed. "It's the only way we'll ever get the miracle we need to fight this plague in Rakai."

❊ ❊ ❊

"How extremely stupid [of me]," Thomas Henry Huxley wrote when he first read *The Origin of Species*, "not to have thought of that!" Convinced by the elegant parsimony of Darwin's description of natural selection's role in evolution, Huxley immediately joined a tight group of scientists defending Darwin from attack and popularizing his work with the public. Darwin called him "my good and admirable agent for the promulgation of damnable heresies"; Huxley's defense of Darwin was so fierce that the press labeled him "Darwin's bulldog."

When Huxley's son Noel died of scarlet fever in September 1860, he channeled his grief into anger at Sir Robert Owen, head of the British Museum's Department of Paleontology, who had published a lengthy, unscrupulous review of *The Origin* in the *Edinburgh Review*. Earlier, Owen had helped Darwin identify some of his fossil specimens from the *Beagle*, including his *Megatherium* skull, but turned coat when he saw that Darwin might unseat him as the scientific pet of London's smart set. Attacking Darwin at the 1860 Oxford meeting of the British Association for the Advancement of Science, Owen claimed he had conclusive proof against application of the theory of evolution to humans. The size and structure of the human brain, he said, was so different from that of any primate it proved that humans could not possibly have descended from the apes.

When the Church of England's Bishop Wilberforce remarked that he would not want an ape for his ancestor, Huxley said, "the Lord hath delivered him into mine hands" as he rose to his feet. "If I would rather have a miserable ape for a grandfather," he said, "or a man highly endowed by nature and possessed of great means and influence, and yet who employs those faculties for the mere purpose of introducing ridicule into a grave scientific discussion—I unhesitatingly affirm my preference for the ape." His verbal slap across the Bishop's face began the duel between fundamentalist Christians and evolutionists that continues to this day.

Darwin's views were remarkably modern, but would await modern genetic analysis for incontrovertible proof. Humans, he argued, were not many species or races, but one because human races "graduate into each other." Academics of his day classified humans into anywhere from three to sixty-three races, but Darwin thought "it is hardly possible to discover clear distinctive characters between them." And these similarities were not just physical. Darwin reported that he had been "incessantly struck, whilst living with the Fuegians on board the 'Beagle,' with the many little traits of character, showing how similar their minds were to ours; and so it was with a full-blooded negro with whom I happened once to be intimate." He referred of course, to John Edmonstone, the freed slave who had been Darwin's "professor" of taxidermy at Edinburgh so many years before.

But controversies among human groups were inevitable. Since "many more individuals are born than can possibly survive," Darwin said, the struggle for existence "almost invariably will be most severe between the individuals of the same species, for they frequent the same districts, require the same food, and are exposed to the same dangers." This competition is so intense that "relatively few members of any species in any generation can emerge as winners." Poet Alfred Lord Tennyson described nature as "red in tooth and claw," but Darwin knew that the workings of evolution are much more subtle, especially for humans. It is impossible to know in advance which variations will be most advantageous in the long term, and while humans can identify those that seem favorable to man, "other variations, useful in some way to each being in the great and complex battle of life, should occur in the course of many successive generations."

As humans, we are "so profound in our ignorance, and so high our presumption," Darwin wrote, that we think we can anticipate evolution's outcomes. It is never possible, he knew, to predict the "many different checks, acting at different periods of life, and during different seasons or years [will] come into play; some one check or some few being generally the most potent; but all will concur in determining the average number or even the existence of the species." AIDS would not have surprised Darwin, a student of Thomas Malthus, but he never would have tried to predict the outcome of this great plague.

※ ※ ※

It was more than a century after Darwin's death in 1882 before the fanaticism surrounding the Social Eugenics movement died down. Generations of people of color have suffered as "experts" tried to determine if one human group or "race" was "better" or "higher" than another. From measuring skull sizes and IQs, to preventing "miscegenation," to outright hanging, to wholesale extermination through war, the weapons of racism are still in use and still know no bounds. Recent findings in molecular genetics that human groups are more alike than different and that all human beings have genetic links to our first African ancestors have so far made little impression.

An uncountable number of atrocities have been perpetrated in the name of medicine and health by "high-minded" people, such as the public health experts behind the Tuskegee Study in the United States, colonial medicine's experiments in segregation and social control, and testing of vaccines and medicines in Africa that are never provided there once they are developed. Cloaked in economic arguments or in arguments for the protection of intellectual property rights, they are perpetrated by people who would deny antiretroviral treatments to people with AIDS who are too poor to pay the exorbitant prices that drug companies demand for the drugs. In the age of AIDS, denial of drugs that keep westerners alive for ten to fifteen years is racism writ large and, to many, nothing short of genocide. As Brazilian AIDS activist Richard Parker says, "vulnerability to HIV and AIDS has increasingly come to be understood as fundamentally linked to questions of social and economic inequality and injustice,"[2] whether they are the questions of cause—why some people get AIDS and some people do not—or questions of effect—who gets treatment and who does not.

Parker orchestrated Brazil's defiance of international trade restrictions and World Bank public health policy to deliver antiretroviral care to all Brazilians. He argues that while the awareness of links between poverty and AIDS was building in the 1990s, the World Bank was gradually defining the HIV/AIDS pandemic in economic terms and linking its management to global capitalist development (globalization) and neoliberal economics. As "the relations between oppression, exploitation, inequality, and HIV infection have become more apparent to us, the global response to the epidemic has simultaneously become more timid," he says. "Today it is the Bank, rather than [the World Health Organization], that issues the most important statements and reports on the status of the epidemic and the policies that should be used for control." The Bank is squeezing humanitarian concern out in favor of cost effectiveness in epidemic control strategies. The tortured deaths of "less valuable" humans can be justified because saving them is not "affordable" or "economically viable."

Through its domination of policy discussions, the World Bank has tried to ensure that the main criteria for evaluating questions of HIV/AIDS policy are economic, not humanitarian. World Bank policymakers have argued, for example, that poor countries should not consider providing treatment to the afflicted and that prevention programs should come first even if people were dying in absolute agony. The same policymakers did not argue that the means to provide care and treatment should be given to countries with large numbers of sufferers, that drug companies should be called to task for letting people die while earning astronomical profits, or that the debts of poor countries should be forgiven so they can "afford" to pay for treatment. Parker reports that in negotiating an AIDS-related loan to Brazil, the policy of antiretroviral distribution became "a major point of contention, classified as it was by the bank as economically irrational and unsustainable."

Brazil finally got the loan, but had to promise it would use none of the proceeds to fund antiretroviral treatment, treatment of opportunistic infections, or care of any type. Brazil's courage in providing treatment despite the World Bank's objections and constant harassment by the United States and the World Trade Organization (WTO) for its manufacture of generic drugs was not only a lifesaver for thousands of Brazilians, it showed the world community that providing treatment drastically cuts new infection rates. Brazil's progressives staunchly defended their right to provide drugs, pointing out that it reduced hospital costs, increased human productivity, extended people's working lives by keeping them well, and reduced the burden on health and social services of long-term illness and death. Darwin persisted with his work in the face of forty-three years of chronic and debilitating illness, and the seven children he did not leave orphaned, give an idea of the possibilities created by treatment. What if his treatments had been viewed as irrational and unsustainable?

To Parker, the World Bank's point of view is fundamentally flawed and unacceptable because "public policy must ultimately stem from discussion and debate of the nature of a good society" and not solely from what makes economic sense. After all, Parker points out, "what any society can afford, whether in military spending or healthcare services, is ultimately a political question about the allocation of resources." Telling poor countries not to take care of their AIDS patients is "just as indefensible as the assertion that the United States (or any similarly well-to-do nations) cannot afford to care for the elderly." The negotiations with the World Bank were seminal in revising Parker's thinking about the relationship between commerce and disease control in the modern world. Although "for political reasons it would never be stated so crudely, the often repeated assertion that AIDS is an exceptionally expensive condition to care for and treat can hardly help but lead to the conclusion that the more rapidly those people living with HIV in the developing world become sick and die, the more 'cost-effective' the response to the epidemic would be." Just like syphilis in the fourteenth century, many people privately believe that AIDS is a way to clear the decks and start the development process all over again.

When economists first modeled the economic loss from AIDS in Africa, they included only the cost of losing skilled labor, not the cost of losing unskilled labor or the unemployed. Costs of treatment in developing countries were not included because, until 2000, treatment was never considered to be a viable option. In evaluating use of antiretrovirals for pregnant women to prevent HIV transmission to their children, an economic model reviewed by Botswanan policymakers said that while the country could afford the treatment to prevent infection of the baby at birth, furnishing treatment to mothers following birth would not be cost effective. Typically shortsighted when it came to measuring the social costs of interventions—as most of these economic models are—the model did not factor in the cost of caring for the children orphaned by the mother's death.

Shameless colonial exploitation of African labor from the 1880s through the 1960s shows us where this kind of economic model originates and how useless a strictly economic point of view is. Globalization is old wine in new bottles, the old book of imperialism and colonialism in a new cover. The intellectual mindset of World Bank–driven international health policy can be traced to the efforts of nineteenth-century colonial powers to control the spread of disease because it threatened their economic well-being. As Parker points out, the "same institutional constellation that gave us the politics of international debt in the 1970s, and structural adjustment in the 1980s, today leads the global fight against an epidemic that its own previous policies did so much to structure."

Global capital wizard George Soros says that markets are "amoral . . . not capable, on their own, of taking care of collective needs such as law and order," providing public goods like healthcare and education, or even paying the costs of their own maintenance. Soros, who became wealthy when he allegedly manipulated the British pound sterling into collapse in the 1980s, says that unrestrained globalization will lead to "very lopsided social development" unless the institutions that protect social concerns are strengthened so they can control it. Neoliberal market economics opposes disease control, education, environmental protection, sanitation, and the provision of social security systems of any type. Globalization and neoliberal economics misallocate public good to private gain, leaving anyone without their own personal safety net marginalized and defenseless.

Developing countries are unable to cope because "the ability of capital to go elsewhere undermines the ability of the state to exercise control over the economy," Soros says. Globalization's creation of market mechanisms without conscience and its ability to move capital out of developing countries are strengthened by organizations like the WTO and render the welfare state that came into existence after World War II "obsolete because the people who require a social safety net cannot leave the country, but the capital the welfare state used to tax can." Developing countries pay the price in growing poverty, disease, and unrest. In April 2000 Cochabamba, Bolivia was wracked by riots to protest rising local water rates. A private, foreign-led consortium dominated by the U.S.-based Bechtel Corporation had taken over the city's water system. As a result, most of the local populace could not afford drinking water. The government had to impose martial law. One commentator wrote that the rebellion in Cochabamba set off "loud alarms, particularly in among the major corporations in the global water business. This business has been booming in recent years—Enron was a big player, before its collapse."

The poor in South America (and many other places) are as short of water as they are of food, while supply of this vital commodity is being turned over to market mechanisms. Experts predict that India will run out of water by the end of the first decade of the century; China is close but will be able to sustain itself for a longer time. Unfortunately, no global agreements have identified the right to drinking water as a fundamental human right. "For the opponents of privatization, who believe that access to clean water *is* a human right," activists believe Cochabamba was an important standoff, sending the message to profiteers that "Third World cities may start refusing to accept deals that put a foreign corporation's hand on the neighborhood pump or household tap. Indeed, water auctions may turn out to test the limits of the global privatization gold rush."

"In our Gilded Age, the poorest of the poor are nearly invisible," writes Columbia University economist Jeffrey Sachs, who has been leading a global rally to assist the poor in AIDS-afflicted countries of Africa. "Seven hundred million people live in the 42 so-called Highly Indebted Poor Countries (HIPCs), where a combination of extreme poverty and financial insolvency marks them for a special kind of despair and economic isolation." While the world's richest countries, The Group of Eight (G8), are moving to provide some debt relief, even if they forgave all debt outright, it would not be enough to raise the poor from degrading, grinding poverty. G8 countries must fund global agencies sufficiently so they can assist HIPC countries to address their "crises of public health, agricultural productivity, environmental degradation, and demographic stress." The world's richest country has been the most unconscientious, irresponsible, and insensitive G8 country of all. "The failure of the United States to pay its UN dues," Sachs says, "is surely the world's most significant default on international obligations, far more egregious than any defaults by impoverished HIPCs."

The United States, WTO, World Bank, and other policymakers they influence are finding it harder and harder to control world debate by ignoring or minimizing public opinion for a number of reasons. First, AIDS is taking bigger and bigger bites out of the economic backbone of so many countries in sub-Saharan Africa that the entire global economy is suffering. The impact on economies will be more severe in countries not providing treatment than in those that are because of the loss of human productivity. Second, human rights activists and humanitarians have leveled the policymaking playing field in a number of ways. Communications innovations over the past twenty years have made it possible for local human rights advocates to link with one another around the globe to insist on the rights of the poor to medicine. Modern communications also facilitate ongoing direct partnerships among churches, charitable organizations, healthcare providers, and individuals in developed countries and their counterparts in African and other developing countries, spreading a new sense of personal connection and responsibility not possible in a world served only by corporate-controlled television.

There are many bright lights in the war against AIDS, and one of the most important may be that it has turned into a rallying ground for the rights of the poor to their fair share of the world's resources. It also has succeeded in making many more people aware that disease is not an "innate fault" but a predetermined outcome for the poor. The wild and uncontrolled spread of the disease also has shown us that "HIV and AIDS are part and parcel of a much broader social and economic configuration in which the processes of globalization, unequal capitalist development, and the politics of health are intertwined" in ways that lead to death, disease, and starvation for billions of people in our world, Parker says.

While economists may be willing to risk that the infection will not move to more "valuable" populations, evolutionary biology suggests that delayed action against HIV/AIDS has produced an enormous reservoir of untamed microbes that are ready to burst forth at any minute and overrun the globe. Thanks to the sense of urgency created by AIDS and the growing capabilities of molecular biology and genetics, we have learned more about the spread of diseases and the relationship between microbes and humans over the past twenty years than we had learned since the late 1800s. The HIV/AIDS epidemic finally has broken the illusion of medicine's control over epidemics and infections, cultivated in public policy thinking since the 1950s. Scientists now are developing a new view of epidemics and of the microbes with which we interact. AIDS has changed our perilously ignorant disrespect for the power of microbes, and our conviction that we could wipe them from the face of the earth has been abruptly changed by AIDS into a more reasonable and humble model of coexistence. Microbes are bugs with which ultimately we must learn how to live, with which we live everyday, and which, in the end, have many positive benefits for us.

History tells us that epidemics last a long, long time. HIV/AIDS will be around for at least the next two or three hundred years, so management policies must keep this in mind. The trajectory of HIV/AIDS growth that started in the late 1980s will continue until the middle of the twenty-first century, with peaks occurring at different times in different places. Then, after a long plateau, there will be a long drop, and AIDS will stabilize worldwide at a lower level and be with us permanently as an endemic, chronic disease. Brazil, Uganda, and Thailand have shown us that we can shorten the time to the peak of the curve if we so choose.

To attack HIV/AIDS, it would be useful to know what conditions of modern living are giving lentiviruses—retroviruses, of which HIV is one, are part of this broad group of slow-acting viruses—the edge. In the United States, autoimmune diseases have become a major cause of death in women of all ages.[3] Multiple sclerosis, lupus, pernicious anemia, myocarditis, chronic hepatitis, and rheumatoid arthritis occur more frequently in women than men and cause the body's immune system to attack its own tissues. AIDS may be part of an overall disease trend, but is spreading faster and farther than other lentiviruses by sex and drugs. Epidemics of venereal disease are among the most damaging, most costly, and most difficult to eradicate. If ordinary epidemics are nature's way of making an "attitude adjustment," violently notching populations down every now and again to better match our planet's carrying capacity, STD epidemics are ongoing safety valves in adaptation that slow population growth by causing infertility. AIDS has blown the discussion of sexuality and disease wide open, and if we have any sense at all as a species, we will come to our senses about the role of sexuality in human affairs.

In the time of AIDS, it is a critical global necessity to stop the nonsense about the immorality of sexual behavior of young people promulgated by religious leaders—particularly annoying from the Catholic church, whose leaders seemed unable to restrain themselves from perpetrating the grossest of criminal acts on their own altar boys—in face of evidence from every corner of the globe to the contrary. Young people need help establishing healthy sex lives in stable family settings, but denying them the means to practice safe sex is as good as condemning them to death in settings with high HIV prevalence. When I managed the U.S. Agency for International Development's countrywide HIV/AIDS program in Tanzania, I traveled to the heart of the country on a review visit, and our vehicle was besieged by young men the minute we came into town. "Where are the condoms?" they wanted to know. "We have not had any for two weeks, and we're not sure we can be celibate much longer!"

Asking for chastity in a world where people's sexual lives diverge markedly from the proscriptions of elite fundamentalists is resulting in rampant growth of the pandemic in fifteen- to twenty-four-year olds. When I was working in Uganda in the early 1990s, Catholic missionaries in the southwestern districts—near Rakai, where Molly, Pauline, and Robina live—were distributing condoms as "necessary health devices," trying to stem the tide of sick and dying demanding their care. While this would not have sat well with the Pope, who was still telling Africans to "go forth and multiply"—these were his words to an audience on his visit to Zimbabwe in 1992—it was a human and caring response in a time of plague offered by experienced and compassionate nuns in defiance of their own pontiff.

The mechanisms and technical means to make responsible family planning a reality for all of the poor in the world exist, but these programs are characteristically underfunded, persecuted by conservatives who have never experienced the desperation of poverty or the despair of HIV infection themselves. Providing the world's desperately poor with the means to control their own reproductive lives will allow humankind to reclaim some of its edge in the world battle against errant microbes. It is shameful that the condom supply to Africa was declining due to lack of donor support just as the growth of HIV/AIDS was increasing perilously fast in eastern and southern Africa in the late 1990s.

In 1975 Edward O. Wilson, after surveying the success of biologists in explaining animal behavior, asked if humans, like animals, are still governed by the primitive instincts garnered in several hundreds of thousand years of evolution on the African savannah. After all, Wilson argued, it has been less than 150,000 years since humans have had language, a few thousand years since humans abandoned hunting and gathering and began living in settled societies, and only a few hundred years since we have had industrialized societies. For only a tiny fraction of the time that we have been on the planet have we even pretended that our minds could help us overcome our instincts. Evolutionary biologists in the 1960s and 1970s documented real consistency of behavior patterns across species,[4] including similarities in male–female relationships and behavior, sexuality, mating, and family composition. Over the past twenty years, evidence accumulated from comparative behavioral studies was confirmed by brain function and genetic research showing specific behavioral coding for specific types of behavior. Research is advancing so quickly on all fronts that it soon may be possible for biologists to link both individual and social behaviors directly to specific genes.

The growing body of evidence that human behavior is conditioned by our evolutionary past has relevance for HIV/AIDS in four ways. First, although our sexual behavior is determined by our genes, how can we change it? Second, can human behavior really be explained by presuming that humans are driven by the desire to maximize the presence of their genes in the next generations, or is it possible that human behavior has become a good deal more subtle than that? Third, if genetic analysis of world populations has revealed two major clusters, "Africans" and "non-Africans," are the centuries of exploitation of Africa by the developed world and the current disinterest in its fate (as measured by the amounts of aid being pledged to the Global AIDS fund and other relief measures) a reflection of this? Finally, how long does it take for human behavior and genetic composition to change in relation to disease?

Sexual behavior, as anyone who has been through the agonies of adolescence can attest, is a remarkably strong and primitive set of instincts that often seem to be beyond conscious control. Yet we also know personally that it is possible to change or control our sexual behavior and that different societies have evolved different patterns of sexual behavior as adaptations to environmental pressures and cultural beliefs. The rise of Calvinism in response to syphilis is one pertinent example, as is the shift in public morality from liberal to conservative during the transition from Regency to Victorian eras, and the shift in the opposite direction from the 1950s into the free love era of the 1960s.

With the HIV/AIDS epidemic it appears that evolution is favoring people who have been and are able to practice caution in their sexual relationships. We saw earlier that the size of the human female body is 80 percent of the male body. Suppose for a minute that this means that 80 percent of all humans have accommodated themselves to relatively safe patterns of sexuality and most of them will never catch HIV. AIDS can take us the rest of the way to monogamy by killing the 20 percent who have not been able to make protective behavior changes voluntarily, or we can choose to supply the support and information that 20 percent need to make positive changes. A large proportion of those 20 percent are young people ages fifteen to twenty-four who are confused about the expression of their sexual needs or are baited into sexual relationships by older people. But when they are given the facts, young people are able, as we have seen, to shift their norms about sex and protect themselves. A young Malawian rap artist advises would-be lovers that "six lovers ain't a mark of manliness but a weakness. . . . Is God unfair y'all it's your own funeral . . . you reap what you sow, that's the whole deal."

AIDS is suggesting that it is prudent to develop new ways to screen desirable mates. Religious organizations in Uganda joined in recommending premarital counseling and HIV screening for young people, and advised

them on safe sex and prevention of mother-to-child transmission. Prospective mates always have had ways to inspect the desirability and health
of their partners. Peacocks have their tail feathers; primitive societies have
mating rituals and proscriptions coded into kinship and family systems.
Some of these are still nearly universal, including taboos against incest and
marrying individuals who are too closely related. Victorians looked for prostitutes and orphans in a family background as signs of instability and lack of
roots. The well-to-do still search family trees, looking for mates who seemed
best able to maintain them in their preferred economic and social status.

If gender relations were taken seriously in HIV/AIDS prevention programs and all other development programs, women could gain control
of their sexuality and exert more control over HIV transmission. In all
known human and nonhuman societies, females are much more conservative
and careful about choosing their mates than males. "Not only do males and
females follow distinct reproductive strategies," says biologist Francis
Fukuyama, "they also respond to different sets of emotional drives. [That is]
why the enjoyment of pornography, like the hiring of prostitutes, is almost
exclusively a male rather than a female pursuit." It probably also explains
why gender equity is so hard to achieve. Why would a male, driven by
entirely different interests, voluntarily cede his control over females? Female
control over their sexuality unquestionably would be useful in HIV/AIDS
prevention, but in many societies women lack even the most basic rights.
Gender bias and partner violence is a kind of terrorism that rules the
everyday lives of billions of women and can no longer be tolerated.

The days following World War II were not only times of anxiety and
tension, says one-time Ford Foundation vice president Francis Sutton, but
times of "optimism and a self-confident readiness to address the new challenge of a global concern with the well-being of human beings, East and
West, North and South."[5] This was the time when all the major human
rights conventions were drafted, guaranteeing the benefits of freedom and
economic justice to all the world's inhabitants. "No longer were there to
be different standards for different races and peoples. Colonialism and 'civilizing missions' were put to an end, and human rights were made universal,"
Sutton says. The UN Declaration of Human Rights made it clear that
"poverty, ignorance, and disease were not to be accepted as our inescapable
mortal lot but to be viewed as evils removable by human effort." This declaration included the responsibility of more developed nations to help those
that were not as well off, a proposition that has been repeatedly affirmed by
international bodies but subsequently ignored by most of the world's developed nations. Globalization and market economics have worked together to

move the world away from its ideals, and the failure of developed countries to keep their commitments is now rearing an ugly, diseased countenance of reproach.

One of the most fundamental violations of human rights is the daily suppression of the rights of half of the world's population, women. As we have seen, denial of women's rights is systematic in developing countries and plays into the hands of the spreading AIDS epidemic. One major international declaration is the Convention on the Elimination of All Forms of Discrimination Against Women (CEDAW), which the United States has persistently refused to ratify despite the promises of Presidents Jimmy Carter and Bill Clinton and despite the fact that, according to Joseph Biden, chair of the Senate Foreign Relations Committee, "for the United States, the treaty will impose a minimal burden." Women in the United States might consider making the ratification of CEDAW the first step in strengthening their global solidarity with women of developing countries, who need the example of forthright policy on women to push the issue in their own countries. Inaction on this issue has been tacitly condoned all over the world; it must stop now if we are to make a dent in the global HIV/AIDS epidemic. Biologist and philosopher C. L. Lewis once said that "man's power over Nature is really the power of some men over other men [and women], with nature as their instrument."

In considering the second question, we know that altruistic behavior is a very real part of animal societies and a very real part of human societies as well.[6] The instinct toward altruism is mirrored in the kinship systems and terminologies of more traditional societies, where biological uncles are considered fathers, and biological cousins are considered sisters and brothers. It has been very difficult for social welfare experts studying the caregiving arrangements and problems of children orphaned by HIV/AIDS to get accurate estimates from villages like Molly's because before AIDS came along, no child was identified as an orphan. British biologist William Hamilton developed the theory of "inclusive fitness" to describe how altruism actually fluctuates among humans in relation to the number of genes they share.

Human behavior, while still conditioned by primitive instincts in some areas, is also determined by more complex genetic coding. Biologists have showed that the ability of humans (and some other species) to create new social rules in response to changing situations is part of our genetic wiring, so that, Fukuyama says "the new biology leaves individual free will and personal responsibility intact; a creature as dependent for survival as man is on learning, intelligence, and consciousness can obviously shape his own destiny to a considerable degree." However, our behavior is not infinitely adaptable; it is limited in ways that also may be genetically coded. Biologist Lionel Trigger says that our emotional structure is geared to a life lived with close kin in small groups, not to the large-scale, crowded, anonymous life of cities. Males of most species are decidedly more violent while females are more inclined to be oriented toward family and children, behaviors that "are rooted in genetics, rather than in a 'sexual identity' that is merely socially constructed. If we fail to adequately socialize young males to non-violence, we are asking for big trouble, a concern in many African countries today where large proportions of young children are orphans.

The third question we must ask with relevance to HIV/AIDS is why Africa, since being "discovered" by the Europeans (and others), has been systematically persecuted, victimized, robbed of its people and its wealth. Is it "genocide by neglect," as some have called the world's failure to respond to HIV/AIDS?[7] Is it, in fact, a case of global apartheid, to borrow the phrase of African scholar and activist Salih Booker? If the rest of the human species is more related to one another than they are related to Africans, is it simply a case that human genetics determines that we suffer less guilt in leaving Africa to fall into ruins? Is this intraspecies rivalry, which, as we learned from Darwin, is the most ruthless of all nature's competitions? If we help Africa, are we helping the "less fit" to survive? Or can we simply assume that the direction of human coevolution with microbes is not necessarily good or beneficial for everyone, as biologist Paul Ewald claims, that nature is indeed red in tooth and claw?

While our attitudes toward Africa may have a genetic basis, we also have been systematically misled in understanding a number of things about Africa critical for us to make clear decisions about right action and social justice. The brutal nature of the slave trade and its devastating impact on African social organization may be known, but is it widely known that forced labor continued almost until independence through labor-exploiting relationships of various kinds, including conscription of Africans to serve Allied forces during both world wars? The brutality of colonial governments exploiting their "pieces" of Africa's "cake" is not a subject widely taught in secondary schools in the West. The fact that colonial governments and postcolonial "partners" did little to prepare their former subjects for independence and fostered new African governments that would follow in their footsteps in exploiting the extractive wealth of the continent is also not well taught. The U.S. government's active support of repressive regimes in Liberia, Zaire, and South Africa responsible for many thousands of deaths is little known, nor is it well known that aid from the United States and other members of the G8 to Africa fell by half in the 1990s, when HIV/AIDS was just taking hold. The terms of globalization have consistently been constructed to deal Africa out of the game, a move that has had extremely deleterious consequences.

The last question relevant to probing the relationship between HIV/AIDS and evolution is the genetic plasticity of humans. How long does evolution take? More specifically, how long does human adaptation to disease take? Many experts have said that human adaptation to HIV/AIDS, our construction of a natural immune response to the virus, is not part of the equation because it takes six or seven generations for an adaptation to develop. The experience of the Nairobi prostitutes and the stabilization of HIV levels in other African populations suggest, however, that this adaptation began some time long ago. It is therefore critical that we act to preserve growth and stability in Africa so that these potential adaptations are maintained, even if we ignore the importance of assisting Africans because they have wider genetic diversity than the other branch of humankind or because we care about all human beings as one. Africans have adaptations to many diseases and a wide array of other genetic traits that could be the basis of a number of disease responses. The very genetic pattern we need to build resistance to HIV/AIDS may be found only in Africa, where the disease first moved from apes to humans.

As Darwin pointed out over a hundred years ago and recent genetic and social research demonstrates, the human body and human social behavior are more complex than any machine or system designed by man, although it has not been produced by deliberate design or control. Biologically simply creatures such as bees, termites, and even bacteria like *Wolbachia*, can produce sophisticated and complex structures and social patterns just by following one or two simple rules. Each of these systems can exist only to the extent that it is adaptive, that it ensures that creatures will survive to the next generation. Each of these systems, as Darwin pointed out, is tied in turn to the success of other creatures—to the web of life, as Darwin called it—in ways that are not obvious and cannot be directly manipulated.

How do any of these questions translate into social action? Biology in particular and science in general is incapable of giving us the answer. "As long as we remain in the realm of science proper," Einstein said, "we never meet with a sentence of the type 'Thou shalt not lie' . . . Scientific statements of facts and relations . . . cannot produce ethical directives." Paul Ewald notes that "because evolutionary changes in disease organisms depend on past, present, and future cultural environments, historians, sociologists, anthropologists, and psychologists need to be involved" in making choices. While science can help us keep pace technologically and conceptually, the decisions lay in our hands. It is critically important that while we deepen our technical appreciation of our coevolutionary relationship with our pathogens and reconceptualize our responses to epidemics on that basis, we deepen our compassion as human beings so the answers to resource allocation decisions enable progress on both fronts.

⌘ ⌘ ⌘

The HIV/AIDS pandemic threatens the well-being of the entire human species in at least five ways. First, in Darwin's words, as nature's potent "check" on global population growth and development, HIV/AIDS brings with it unprecedented illness, suffering, and death, distorting population distribution and structures. Our failure to contain population growth over the past two centuries has exceeded the land's carrying capacity. World population has grown from a little more than 1 billion in 1850 to 6 billion at the close of the twentieth century, and will reach 10 billion by 2100. The resulting crowding and resource shortages are exacerbated by a global economic system that keeps billions of people hanging on to life by their fingernails while only the very few can prosper. Laissez-faire capitalism has triumphed in the guise of neoliberal market economics. Populations everywhere are exceeding the carrying capacity of both their agricultural systems and their water supplies, struggling to keep up with demands of developed countries that are consuming their capital resources to sustain elaborate modern lifestyles. Unchecked disease is the result.

Second, the global extraction system is having the same impact on Africa as colonial demands for resources in the nineteenth and twentieth centuries. Famine and disease follow one another in cycles because the population never gets strong enough to develop the systems needed for defense; in fact, health and education systems have been corroded by world economic policies in the 1990s. Famine is raging again across southern Africa, taking millions to the edge of starvation, and the cause is only partially HIV/AIDS. Pushing populations to the brink of death and self-control creates multiple security concerns, both for those populations and us, but HIV/AIDS is a security concern that transcends the chaos and collapse of a few countries in Africa. It will go on to upset the security of some very large countries in Asia that are key players in the global economy. While Africans do not have the means to insist on justice, the political response of large Asian have-not countries that have weapons of mass destruction is harder to predict. While the world's rich may not voluntarily decide to share resources with the poor through mechanisms like the Global Fund on AIDS, the game may be forced through other means. No matter how many epidemiologists the Central Intelligence Agency hires, it cannot predict the effects of widespread epidemics. As Malcolm Gladwell says in *The Tipping Point*, "a world that follows the rules of epidemics is a very different place from the world we think we live in now." In that world, things happen a lot faster and totally out of proportion to the way they happen in a normal world.

Third, HIV/AIDS has already created a decided global economic drag, a downward spiral of lost productivity, increasing numbers of sick and vulnerable, and soaring costs of healthcare that threaten our markets, our producers, and our pocketbooks. The drag will become much, much worse by the end of this decade in Africa and will become especially critical when Asian countries begin to experience more widespread illness and death. Africa will lose an estimated 20 percent of its population productivity by 2010, and Asia is likely to experience the same magnitude of loss between 2010 and 2020. Globalization means that the prosperity of developed countries depends on cheap production and growing markets in developing countries; widespread illness and death means they will disappear. And then there is the cost of care if the developed world decides to help, a precaution that may be self-defensive in a world of interconnected microbes.

Fourth, HIV/AIDS has created a huge and ever-growing disease reservoir that now numbers 40 million people and is likely to exceed 110 million by the end of the decade. The existence of this reservoir is fundamentally dangerous to the developed world in light of our limited knowledge of the disease and our limited ability to predict how it may increase in virulence and mutate as its reservoir grows. And as HIV/AIDS joins the existing disease reservoir, there is a real possibility that it could combine with malaria, tuberculosis, cholera, and other killers. This effect is more likely if we provide treatment only for richer sufferers, because virulence will increase as the life spans of disease carriers shortens.

As Joshua Lederburg says, "most people are grossly overoptimistic with respect to the means we have available to forfend global epidemics comparable to the Black Death of the fourteenth century.... We are complacent to trust that nature is benign; we are arrogant to assert that we have the means to except ourselves from the competition." As this enormous reservoir of infection steadily grows, the global public health system, the early warning system and first line of defense against the spread of plagues from developing to developed countries, is breaking down. The ability of diseases literally to fly around the world undetected makes them much more efficient than any terrorist network.[8] WHO's new rapid response unit was established in 1996 to improve the containment of deadly disease outbreaks, but it is having trouble getting funding from developed member countries. When we consider the spread of syphilis in the fourteenth century, before the age of globalization, we must wonder how well emerging diseases will be contained.

Finally, HIV/AIDS creates a permanent reservoir of shame in developed countries. In the face of an epidemic, failure to act is a form of action on the part of those who are not infected. Throughout the 1990s, U.S. funding for HIV prevention in developing countries averaged some $70 million per year, about the same as the U.S. military allocated for Viagra when this medication first became available. Although the United States is the largest donor in the world for HIV/AIDS programs, $70 million is paltry when compared to the $10 billion per year experts say is needed over the next ten years to control HIV/AIDS in Africa alone. In the two years since its optimistic and much-heralded establishment as a funding mechanism for relatively painless transfer of the resources needed from rich countries to poor, the Global Fund for AIDS has gained $2 billion in pledges of the $10 billion per year needed and only $1 billion had been received by July 2002. By June 2003, lack of pledges threatened to put the Fund out of business. We continue to lose vital time in addressing and controlling the growth of the reservoir, considering that viral time lines for mutation and resistance are very, very short.

More shameful still is the fact that the total amount African nations pay for debt service each year, $14.5 billion, is greater than the total aid they receive, resulting in a net outflow each year from the poorest of the world's poor into the pockets of the rich. Debt service represents 5 percent of the gross domestic product and 15 percent of export earnings of African countries.[9] The poor are, in fact, paying us each year, with the absolute result that millions in Africa exist on the edge of starvation. African governments are hamstrung by their debt, paying out millions of dollars in debt service that they have pledged to spend on health and AIDS prevention if they receive debt relief.

Nigeria, with one of the largest national populations on the subcontinent and its HIV/AIDS epidemic poised for rapid take-off, has been struggling to pay off a national debt of $33 billion (93 percent of its gross national product) for almost five years. Most of the debts were incurred by a corrupt military government whose members sold oil concessions in the country and kept the money for themselves. Since ending military rule in 1999, Nigeria's leaders have tried to negotiate debt relief, arguing that under current lending conditions the country will pay five dollars for every dollar owed by 2010. In 2001 then British high commissioner to Nigeria Philip Thomas told a press conference that since many of the projects financed by international lending failed, foreign creditors, including individual countries and the

World Bank, must take responsibility for their bad recommendations. However, the International Monetary Fund (IMF) has declared Nigeria ineligible for debt relief because of its oil resources, overlooking the fact that when oil companies stopped producing in the country in September 2002, it was unable to service its external debts. Nigeria has repeatedly begged for debt relief but has only been forgiven 4 percent of the total stock. Canada retired 1 percent in 1990, and the United States, which gets 10 percent of its oil from Nigeria, forgave its 3 percent of the total—about $10 million, roughly the same amount it cancelled for Egypt and Poland in 1991. Other creditors refuse to budge.

HIV/AIDS and declining agricultural production are now in a negative synergistic relationship, creating the need for more and faster debt relief. Half of Africa's children are already moderately or seriously malnourished, and the number is getting worse each year. This kind of malnutrition not only results in permanent cognitive damage and failure of mental development, but makes the poor more susceptible to infections of all kinds, including HIV/AIDS. It makes treatment for AIDS impossible, because drugs must be taken with food.

The raging AIDS pandemic in sub-Saharan Africa, which will have striking and irreversible consequences for the human species, is a direct result of global neglect of a continent viewed by many as in irreparable chaos, with little remaining economic, strategic, or market relevance to leading global interests. The terrible global consequences of this humanitarian crisis, unprecedented in the modern world, can best be understood with reference to the history of the HIV/AIDS pandemic itself, to marginalization and mismanagement by the international authorities charged with its control, and with reference to past epidemics. It can be addressed only if its relevance for the continuity of the development, health, and genetic diversity of the human species and the threat of slowdown of global economic growth, future prosperity, and global stability is recognized. As Brazil's Richard Parker has demonstrated, AIDS is clearly another manifestation of global processes gone wrong, neoliberal economists hijacking the public's health from the ethical and public arena. The economic success of Brazil's defiance of economic "logic" to provide treatment demonstrates that humanitarian concern can drive good decision making in the global arena.

The well of shame is growing deeper with each day of neglect, each day when some 5,000 more dead from AIDS are buried, most of them in Africa. It may be no accident that one of most pressing health problems in the United States is depression and that our children are increasingly prone to suicide and violence. Shame and guilt are very difficult burdens to bear.

Boys like David and Douglas, who are the miracle of Africa, have the right to an opportunity to grow from modeling orchestras and marching bands in mud to making exquisite pieces of art in paint, clay, or stone or to lead marching bands of their own. We must hurry so that their capacity, like Darwin's, is not lost to disease, that they do not become pitiful, unidentified markers on a pile of stones in a lonely banana grove. This decision could be the miracle of the world.

Asunta Wagura, a member of the Kenya Network of Women with AIDS is one of the 30 million or so individuals alive in Africa today who is struggling with the virus. She demands her due from us, asserting her right to be a partner and not just a victim. "So," she says. "Here I am, an ordinary person with what is rapidly becoming a most ordinary virus. I have stopped feeling sorry for myself and I have now learned to live, think and even act positively. I have come out of my hideout, and I have found a stage where I can tell the world over that I am not a victim but rather I am a messenger. A messenger of hope.... Tell me I am not a number, a statistic, but an equal partner in this struggle."

American novelist John Steinbeck once said, "we have usurped many of the powers we once ascribed to God. Fearful and unprepared, we have assumed lordship over the life and death of the whole world of living things. The danger and the glory and the choice rest finally in man. The test of his perfectibility is at hand... having taken God-like power, we must seek in ourselves for the responsibility and the wisdom we once prayed some deity might have. Man himself has become our greatest hazard and our only hope."

Notes

CHAPTER 1

1. *Matooke* is the Ugandan staple food, a fibrous, fresh-tasting cooking banana that resembles plantain. Steamed and mashed, it is served with "soups" of broth, fish, offal (animal intestines), or vegetables.
2. Molly, Pauline and Robina's story has been fictionalized from real community activities in Uganda's Rakai District in 1989, combined with community stories from other countries that I have witnessed while working in Africa from 1989 to 2001. While a few of the characters are based on real people, many of the events and all of the dialogue have been invented. None of the opinions expressed can be attributed to actual people.
3. "Slim Disease" was the nickname Ugandans gave to AIDS because the diarrhea it caused led to such extensive wasting in most early victims that they quickly became skeletal in appearance. Most patients also developed Kaposi's sarcoma, a skin cancer that causes black skin lesions all over the body.
4. Ankoles and Bugandas are two of the most common tribes in Uganda.
5. Sources for Darwin's story in this and subsequent chapters include J. Browne, *Charles Darwin: Voyaging*, v. 1, and Browne, *Charles Darwin: A Sense of Place*, v. 2 (New York: Knopf, 1995 and 2002); C. Darwin, *The Voyage of the Beagle* (New York: Collier, 1937); C. Darwin, *The Origin of the Species By Means of Natural Selection or The Preservation of Favored Races in the Struggle for Life* (New York: The Modern Library, 1993); and C. Darwin, *The Descent of Man and Selection in Relation to Sex* (New York: Collier Books, 1962); W. Karp, *Charles Darwin and the Origin of the Species* (New York: Harper & Row, 1968); P. Singer, *A Darwinian Left: Politics, Evolution and Cooperation* (New Haven, CT: Yale University Press, 1999).
6. See page 5 of the April 2003 *National Geographic* for a picture of this giant Jurassic period sloth.
7. D. Morens, "Certain Diseases, Uncertain Explanations," *Science*, v. 294 (2001), pp. 1658–1659.
8. T. McMichael, *Human Frontiers, Environments, and Disease: Past Patterns, Uncertain Futures* (Cambridge: Cambridge University Press, 2002), p. 28.
9. T. McMichael, 2002, p. 27.
10. S. Davis, *Reservoirs of Men: A History of the Black Troops of French West Africa* (Westport, CT: Negro Universities Press, 1934), p. 165. Jamaican-born Marcus

Garvey, also called the "Black Moses," led the multi-country "Back to Africa" movement in the early 1900s. He founded the Universal Negro Improvement Association, which was based in his adopted Harlem from 1916 until his indictment for mail fraud in 1922. Deported as an undesirable alien by U.S. president Calvin Coolidge in 1927, he died in relative obscurity in London in 1940.

11. UNAIDS, 2002, "AIDS Epidemic Update," (Geneva, December 2002), p. 29.
12. J. Lederberg, "Pandemic as a Natural Evolutionary Phenomenon," in M. Arien, ed., *In Time of Plague: The History and Consequences of Lethal Epidemic Disease* (New York: New York University Press, 1991), pp. 35–36.

CHAPTER 2

1. Oral thrush, or candidiasis, is a common opportunistic infection that first produces harmless white or red spots of fungus on the tongue, gums, cheek linings, and throat, but can block bronchial airways unless it is treated with an antifungal.
2. Philly Bongoley Lutaaya's "Alone and Afraid" CD was sponsored by the Swedish Red Cross and can still be purchased on the web. Two videos about his life— "Born in Africa" (the title of one of his most popular songs), made in Uganda as he was dying, and "The Legacy of Philly Lutaaya"—still inspire Africans in many countries.
3. American Public Health Association, *The Nation's Health*, 28, no. 4 (April 1998), p. 1 and "AIDS, STDs continue to hit hard in southern United States," *The Nation's Health*, June/July 2003, p. 9.
4. Sources for AIDS include UNAIDS, the 2002 *Report on the Global HIV/AIDS Epidemic* and the 2001 "AIDS Epidemic Update," (December 2001), both of which can be accessed at www.unaids.org. Also see the World Health Organization, *The World Health Report 2001* (WHO: Geneva, 2002); K. DeCock et al., "Shadow on the Continent: Public Health and HIV/AIDS in Africa in the 21st Century," Lancet, v. 360, i. 9326 (July 6, 2002); M. Merson, J. Dayton, and K. O'Reilly, "Effectiveness of HIV Prevention Interventions in Developing Countries," *AIDS*, v. 14, Supplement 2 (2002), pp. 68–84; "What Factors Affect the Prevalence of HIV in Sub-Saharan Africa?" *Population Briefs: Reports on Population Council Research*, 8, no. 1 (2002), p. 1; A. Vakhovskiy, "Winning the War on AIDS, Brazil Style," *Dartmouth Free Press* (August 10, 2001); "Hope for the Best. Prepare for the Worst," *The Economist* (July 13, 2002), pp. 66–67; J. Caldwell, P. Caldwell, and P. Quiggin, "The Social Context of AIDS in Sub-Saharan Africa," pp. 185–234, and J. Caldwell, P. Caldwell, and I. O. Orubuloye, "The Family and Sexual Networking in Sub-Saharan Africa: Historical Regional Differences and Present-day Implications," in Health Transition Special Series No. 4, *Sexual Networking and AIDS in Sub-Saharan Africa: Behavioural Research and the Social Context* (Australian National

University Health Transition Center, 1994), pp. 172–193; UN Fund for Population Activities, "Advances in New Technologies and Issues, Male Circumcision," *Strategic Guidance on HIV Prevention* (UNFPA: New York, 2003, or www.unfpa.org/hiv/strategic/); B. Boyle, "South Africa Prepares Reversal on AIDS Therapy," Reuters (April 28, 2002); M. Ainsworth and W. Teokul, "Breaking the Silence: Setting Realistic Priorities for AIDS Control in Less-Developed Countries," *The Lancet*, 356 (2002), pp. 55–60; P. Alagiri et al., "Global Spending on HIV/AIDS in Resource-Poor Settings," part 3 of *Spending on the HIV/AIDS Epidemic*, Kaiser Family Foundation and Ford Foundation (2002, www.kff.org); S. Ramsay, "Global Fund Makes Historic First Round of Payments," *The Lancet*, 359 (May 4, 2002), p. 6; P. Bergin, "Conservationists Encourage Increased Spending for AIDS in Africa," African Wildlife Foundation press release (February 28, 2003); J. Laurence, "It Isn't Over," *AIDS Patient Care and STDs*, v. 12, no. 1 (1998), pp. 3–4; J. McGeary, "Death Stalks a Continent: In the Dry Timber of African Societies, AIDS Was a Spark," *Time Magazine*, 157, no. 6 (2001), p. 36; K. Stanecki, *The AIDS Pandemic in the 21st Century* (www.usaid.gov/pop_health/aids/publications); UNAIDS, UNICEF, USAID, *Children on the Brink 2002: A Joint Report on Orphan Estimates and Program Strategies* (Washington, DC: TvT Associates/The Synergy Project, 2002 at www.synergyaids.org); M. Greene, "What Will Become of Africa's AIDS Orphans?," *The New York Times Magazine* (December 22, 2002), pp. 49–55; World Bank, *Education and HIV/AIDS: A Window of Hope* (Washington, DC: World Bank, 2002 or www.worldbank.org/hiv_aids/publications); UNFPA, "HIV/AIDS and Poverty," *State of the World's Population* (New York: UNFPA, 2002 or www.unfpa.org); Food and Agriculture Organization, "HIV/AIDS Devastating Rural Labour Force in Many African Countries," Rome (press release January 30, 2001 or www.fao.org/archives); "ILO Says HIV/AIDS Impact on African Development 'Underestimated,'" Rome: International Labour Organization (press release July 11, 2002 or www.ilo.org); American Public Health Association, "HIV/AIDS worsens hunger crisis in southern African countries," *The Nation's Health*, (November 2002), p. 12; R. Swarns, "Meager Harvests in Africa Leave Millions at the Edge of Starvation," *The New York Times* (June 23, 2002), p. 1; S. Booker, "IMF and the World Bank Blamed for Worst Health Crisis in History," *Foreign Policy in Focus* (May 16, 2002, at www.fpif.org); "SA Cemetery Crisis," *African Business* (April, 2002), p. 6; American Public Health Association, "AIDS, STDs continue to hit hard in southern United States," *The Nation's Health* (June/July, 2003), p. 9.

5. D. Gordon et al., "The Next Wave of HIV/AIDS: Nigeria, Ethiopia, Russia, India and China" (Washington, DC: National Intelligence Council, September, 2002), ICA 2002–04D; M. Specter, "India's Plague," *The New Yorker* (December 17, 2001), pp. 74–85.

6. L. Garrett, "Amplification," in R. DeSalle, ed., *Epidemic! The World of Infectious Disease* (New York: New Press, 1999), p. 193.

7. M. White, "Source List and Detailed Death Tolls for the Twentieth Century Hemoclysm," 2002, at www.wusers.erols.com/mwhite28/warstat1.htm; White is also the source for death toll information cited in the remainder of this paragraph. He compares estimates from a wide variety of sources to increase reliability.

8. N. Eberstadt, "The Future of AIDS," *Foreign Affairs*, 81, no. 6 (2002), pp. 22–45.

9. References on migration include A. Kroeber, "The Hot Zone," *Wired* (November 2002), pp. 201–205; J. Wojcicki, " 'She Drank His Money': Survival Sex and the Problem of Violence in Taverns in Gauteng Province, South Africa," *Medical Anthropological Quarterly*, 16, no. 3 (2002), pp. 267–293; B. Ehrenreich and A. Hochschild, eds., *Global Woman: Nannies, Maids and Sex Workers in the New Economy* (New York: Metropolitan Books, 2002); S. Chantavanich et al., *Mobility and HIV/AIDS in the Greater Mekong Subregion* (Bangkok: Asian Development Bank and United Nations Development Program, 2000 or www.adb.org); K. Jochelson, *The Colour of Disease: Syphilis and Racism in South Africa, 1880–1950* (New York: Palgrave, 2001); T. Sowell, *Migrations and Cultures: A World View* (New York: Basic Books, 1996); S. Rajagopalan and R. Nagarajan, "Nurses, Teachers Chasing the American Dream," *Sunday Hindustan Times* (New Delhi, India, February 16, 2003); UN Population Division, *International Migration Report 2002* (New York: UN Publications, 2002); World Tourism Organization, *Tourism Highlights 2002* (Madrid: World Tourism Organization, 2002).

10. H. Epstein, "The Hidden Cause of AIDS," *The New York Review* (May 9, 2002), pp. 43–49.

11. R. Shilts, *And the Band Played On: Politics, People and the AIDS Epidemic* (New York: St. Martin's Press, 1987), p. 83.

12. J. Hirsch et al., "The Social Construction of Sexuality: Marital Infidelity and Sexually Transmitted Disease—HIV Risk in a Mexican Migrant Community," *American Journal of Public Health*, 92, no. 8 (2002), pp. 1227–1237.

13. AIDS and armies are the subject of K. Key, "Soldiers March Home with New Specter of Death," *Infectious Disease Weekly* (July 17, 1995), pp. 11–13; and H. Cauvin, "Stability of Africa Is Threatened as AIDS Gets Foothold in Armies," *New York Times*, International Edition (November 24, 2002), pp. 1–12.

14. For street children, see the Kaiser Daily HIV/AIDS Report (May 28, 2002, www.kff.org); N. Ansell and L. Young, "Young AIDS Migrants in Southern Africa," British Department for International Development, DFID Contract R 7896 or www.dfid.gov.uk (2003); C. Lockhart, "*Kunyenga*, 'Real Sex,' and Survival," *Medical Anthropological Quarterly*, 16, no. 3 (2003), pp. 294–311; Stephens, A., "AIDS Becomes a National Security Issue, *National Journal* (November 18, 2000), p. 3680.

15. Poverty references include D. Narayan and G. Pennushi, *Poverty Trends and Voices of the Poor* (Washington, DC: World Bank Poverty Reduction and

Economic Management Group, 1999 or www.worldbank.org); R. Parker, "The Global HIV/AIDS Pandemic, Structural Inequalities, and the Politics of International Health, *American Journal of Public Health*, 92, no. 3 (2002), pp. 343–346; D. Bloom et al., "AIDS & Economics," Working Group 1, WHO Commission on Macroecnoomics and Health (Geneva: World Health Organization, 2001 or www.cmhealth.org/cmh_popapers&reports.htp); UNDP, *Human Development Report* (New York: UN Development Program, 1998); C. Blackden and C. Bhanu, *Gender, Growth, and Poverty Reduction: Special Program of Assistance for Africa*, 1998 Status Report on Poverty (World Bank Poverty Technical Working Group Paper No. 428, www.addall.com, 1998);

16. H. Epstein, 2002, p. 48.
17. Condom material comes from "Birth Control," *Encyclopaedia Britannica*, v. 15 (Macropedia 2002 edition, 2002), pp. 113–114; Averting HIV&AIDS, "Condoms: History, Effectiveness, and Testing," (www.avert.org, 2002); J. Fowles, "Notes on the History of the Condom," Planned Parenthood Federation of America (2002, www.plannedparenthood.org); D. Nelkin and S. Gilman, "Placing the Blame for Devastating Disease," in M. Arien, M., ed., *In Time of Plague: The History and Consequences of Lethal Epidemic Disease* (New York: New York University Press, 1991), pp. 39–56.
18. J. Badger, "Worldwide Male Circumcision Rates," (2003, at www.circlist.com/rites/rates/html).
19. For drug access and vaccines, see World Trade Organization, "TRIPS: Counsel Discussion on Access to Medicines, Developing Country Group's Paper," (June 19, 2001 at www.wto.org); K. Baldwin, "Latin American AIDS Activists Turn on Brazil," Reuters (May 25, 2002); SRI Media, "HIV/AIDS: TRIPPS and President Bush's 'Emergency Plan for AIDS Relief'" (February 11, 2003, www.srimedia.com); World Health Organization and World Trade Organization, *WTO Agreements and Public Health*, (2002, www.wto.org); O. Jablonski, "Accelerating Access: Serving Pharmaceutical Companies and Corrupting Health Systems," (Act Up-Paris, May 14, 2002); S. Gottlieb, "Drug Companies Maintain 'Astounding' Profits," *British Medical Journal*, May 4, 2002 at www.bmj.com/cgi/contents/full); SRI Media, "AIDS Drug Will Cost Each Patient $20,000 a Year" (February 24, 2003, www.srimedia.com); R. Carroll, "African's AIDS drugs trapped in the laboratory: Kenya has the pills. Now the fight is on to get them to the people," *The Guardian* (May 21, 2003), p. NA; M. Specter, "The Vaccine," *The New Yorker* (February 3, 2003), pp. 54–65; SRI Media, "AIDS Vaccine Dramatic Findings," (February 24, 2003, www.srimedia.com); J. Cohen, "Malawi: A Suitable Case for Treatment," *Science*, v. 297 (August 9, 2002), pp. 927–929.
20. M. Wilson, *A World Guide to Infections: Diseases, Distribution, Diagnosis* (New York: Oxford University Press, 1991), pp. 6–8.
21. In addition to World Health Organization, UNAIDS includes the United Nations Children's Fund (UNICEF); United Nations Development Program

(UNDP); United Nations Fund for Population Activities (UNFPA); United
Nations Educational, Scientific, and Cultural Organization (UNESCO);
United Nations Drug Control Program (UNDCP); the World Bank; the
International Labor Organization (ILO); and the Food and Agricultural
Organization (FAO).

22. For virus mechanics, see L. Garrett, *The Coming Plague* (New York: Farrar,
Straus and Giroux, 1994); N. Boyce, "New Plagues of Monkey Viruses?" *U.S.
News and World Report* (April 8, 2002), p. 56; A. Fettner, *Viruses: Agents of
Change* (New York: McGraw-Hill, 1990); K. Bellenir and P. Dresser, eds., *AIDS
Sourcebook*, Health Reference Series, v. 4 (Detroit, MI: Omnigraphics, Inc.,
1995); D. Ward, *The AmFAR AIDS Handbook: The Complete Guide to
Understanding HIV and AIDS* (New York: W. W. Norton and Company, 1999);
M. Klesius, "Search for a Cure," *National Geographic* (February 2002),
pp. 32–43; G. Garnett and E. Holmes, "The Ecology of Emergent Infectious
Disease," *BioScience*, 46, no. 2 (1996), pp. 127–136; C. Zimmer, *Evolution: The
Triumph of an Idea* (New York: HarperCollins, 2001).

23. For behavior, see Centers for Disease Control, "Study Indicates Americans Place
Themselves at Risk," *Morbidity and Mortality Weekly Review* (March 24, 2002),
p. 22; B. Crossette, "U.N. Finds AIDS Knowledge Still Lags in Stricken
Nations," *The New York Times* (June 23, 2002), p. 10; S. Dube, *Sex, Lies and
AIDS* (New Delhi: HarperCollins India, 2000); M. Seshu and J. Csete, "India's
Voiceless Women Are Easy Prey for AIDS," *Los Angeles Times* (December 1,
2002); "Research Shows that United States may be due for resurgent HIV epi-
demic," *AIDS Alert*, v. 16, no.10 (October, 2001), p. 121; S. Chen et. al.,
"Continuing Increases in Sexual Risk Behavior and Sexually Transmitted
Diseases Among Men Who Have Sex with Men," *American Journal of Public
Health*, v. 92, no. 9 (September, 2002), p. 1387; American Public Health
Association, "Life expectancy increases overall, drops for blacks," *The Nation's
Health* (May, 2003), p. 21; S. Maman et al., "HIV-Positive Women Report
More Lifetime Partner Violence," *American Journal of Public Health*, 92, no. 9
(2002), pp. 1331–1337; "CDC Reports the Health-Related Costs of Intimate
Partner Violence Against Women Exceeds $5.8 billion each year in the United
States," (press release, Atlanta, GA: Centers for Disease Control, www.cdc.gov);
L. Van Gelder, "The Beauty of Health: AIDS," *Ms. Magazine* (May 1983),
p. 1–3; E. Brown, "Crystal Ball," *New York* (April 29, 2002), pp. 35–37; J. Levi,
"Ensuring Timely Access to Care for People with HIV Infection: A Public
Health Imperative," *American Journal of Public Health*, 92, no. 3 (2002),
pp. 339–340; G. Herek et al., "HIV-Related Stigma and Knowledge in the
United States: Prevalence and Trends, 1991–1999," *American Journal of Public
Health*, 92, no. 3 (2002), pp. 371–377; M. Burford, "Girls and Sex: You Won't
Believe What's Going On," *O Magazine* (November, 2002), pp. 212–215;
K. Mojidi, "Repositioning Family Planning in Africa: A Call to Action,"
USAID in Africa (Fall 2002), p. 7; D. Carr et al., *Youth in Sub-Saharan*

Africa: A Chartbook on Sexual Experience and Reproductive Health (Washington, DC: Macro International, 2001); M. Lytle,"Better Prostitution Through Technology," *Wired* (December 2002), p. 38; M. Gladwell, *The Tipping Point: How Little Things Can Make a Big Difference* (Boston: Little, Brown, 1998), chapter 7; American Public Health Association, "Substance Abuse, Alcohol Linked to Unprotected Sex," *The Nation's Health* (April 2002), p. 15; C. Wright, "Programs Don't Affect Teens' Sexual Activity," *The Nation's Health* (December 2002/January 2003), p. 21; UNAIDS, *A Measure of Success in Uganda: The Value of Monitoring Both HIV Prevalence and Sexual Behavior* (Geneva: UNAIDS, May 1998; www.unaids.org/publications); UNICEF, UNAIDS, and WHO, *Young People and HIV/AIDS: Opportunity in Crisis*, (www.unaids.org/ publications, 2002); U.S. Census Bureau, *World Population Profiles 1994 and 1996* (www.census.gov/publications, 1994 and 1996).

24. H. Miletski, *Understanding Bestiality and Zoophila*, (Bethesda, MD: East-West Publishing Company, 2002), p. 61; D. Beers, "You Sexy Animal, You," (Alternet.org, 2002); A. Fausto-Sterling, "Why Do We Know So Little About Human Sex?" *Discover* (June 1992), pp. 28–30.

CHAPTER 3

1. A potent distilled spirit made from banana that tastes like gin with the lime already in it.
2. References on African development include P. Schwab, *Africa: A Continent Self-Destructs* (New York: Palgrave, 2001); D. Bloom and J. Sachs, "Geography, Demography, and Economic Growth in Africa," *Brookings Papers on Economic Activity*, issue 2 (1998), pp. 207–295; N. Chazan et al., *Politics and Society in Contemporary Africa*, 3rd ed. (Boulder, CO: Lynne Rienner Publishers, 1999); K. Jochelson, *The Colour of Disease* (London: Palgrave, 2001); Global Policy Forum, "Nile River Politics: Who Receives Water?" (August 10, 2000, www.globalpolicy.org/security/natres/nile.htm); D. Leonard and S. Straus, *Africa's Stalled Development: International Causes and Cures* (Boulder, CO: Lynne Rienner Publishers, 2003); A. Cowell, "40 Nations in Accord on 'Conflict Diamonds,'" *New York Times* (November 6, 2002), p. 5; R. Monastersky, "Stemming the Flow of Blood Diamonds," *Chronicle of Higher Education*, 48, no. 44 (July 12, 2002), p. A18; "A Bloody Trade: Big Diamond Companies Hold the Key to Halting Illegal Mining," *New Scientist*, v. 174, no. 2344 (May 25, 2002), p. 5; J. Anderson, "Our New Best Friend," *The New Yorker* (October 7, 2002), pp. 74–83; G. Ayittey, *Africa Betrayed* (New York: St. Martin's Press, 1992); G. Ayittey, *Africa in Chaos* (New York: St. Martin's Press, 1998); "International Relations," *Encyclopaedia Britannica*, v. 21 (2002); J. Diamond, *Guns, Germs and Steel: The Fates of Human Societies* (New York: W. W. Norton and Company, 1997).

3. S. Watts, *Epidemics and History: Disease, Power and Imperialism* (New Haven, CT: Yale University Press, 1997), p. 109. For slavery, also see N. Chazan, P. Schwab; L. Henderson, *Angola: Five Centuries of Conflict* (Ithaca, NY: Cornell University Press, 1979); B. Davidson, *The African Slave Trade: Pre-Colonial History 1450–1850* (Boston: Little, Brown, 1961).

4. For information on labor conscription during World War I and II, see J. Ashley, "South African Soldiers and Defence," *Journal of Southern African Studies*, v. 22, no. 3 (2003), p. 505; A. Clayton, *France, Soldiers and Africa* (London: Brassey's Defence Publishers/Pergamon, 1988); S. Davis, *Reservoirs of Men: A History of the Black Troops of French West Africa* (Westport, CT: Negro Universities Press, 1934); M. Echenberg, *Colonial Conscripts: The Tirailleurs Sénégalais in French West Africa 1857–1960* (Portsmouth, NH: Heinemann, 1991); J. Foltz and H. Bienen, *Arms and the African: Military Influence on Africa's International Relations* (New Haven, CT: Yale University Press, 1985); A. Jackson, "African Soldiers and Imperial Authorities: Tensions and Unrest During the Service of High Commission Territories Soldiers in the British Army, 1941–46," *Journal of Southern African Studies*, v. 25, no. 4 (1999), pp. 645–666; N. Lawler, *Soldiers of Misfortune: Ivoirien Tirailleurs of World War II* (Athens: Ohio University Press, 1992); J. Lunn, *Memoirs of the Maelstrom: A Senegalese Oral History of the First World War* (Portsmouth, NH: Heinemann, 1999); " 'Les Races Geurrieres': Racial Preconceptions in the French Military about French West African Soldiers during the First World War," *Journal of Contemporary History*, v. 34, no. 4 (1999), p. 517–536; H. Moyse-Bartlett, *The King's African Rifles* (London: Gale & Polden, 1956); M. Page, "Malawians in the Great War and After, 1914–1925," Ph.D. dissertation (Department of History, Michigan State University, 1977); T. Parsons, *The African Rank-and-File: Social Implications of Colonial Military Service in the King's African Rifles, 1902–1964* (Portsmouth, NH: Heinemann, 1999); A. Summers and R. Johnson, "World War I Conscription and Social Change in Guinea," *Journal of African History*, v. 29, no. 1 (1978), pp. 25–38; M. Thompson, "Colonial Policy and the Family Life of Black Troops in French West Africa, 1817–1904," *International Journal of African Historical Studies*, v. 23, no. 3 (1990), pp. 423–453.

5. References on postcolonial Africa include B. Freud, *The Making of Contemporary Africa: The Development of African Society Since 1800* (Boulder, CO: Lynne Rienner Publishers, 1998), p. 170; N. Chazan; Kingsolver, B., *The Poisonwood Bible* (New York: Harper & Row, 1998).

6. For social history, see J. Iliffe, *The African Poor: A History* (New York: Cambridge University Press, 1987). For an excellent review African social organization and its relationship to the spread of HIV/AIDS, see J. Caldwell, P. Caldwell, and P. Quiggin, "The Social Context of AIDS in Sub-Saharan Africa," pp. 129–162, and J. Caldwell, P. Caldwell, and I. O. Orubuloye, "The Family and Sexual Networking in Sub-Saharan Africa: Historical Regional Differences and Present-Day Implications," in Health Transition Special Series No. 4, *Sexual Networking*

and AIDS in Sub-Saharan Africa: Behavioural Research and the Social Context (Australian National University Health Transition Center, 1994), pp. 171–194.

CHAPTER 4

1. For information on diseases, see C. Turkington and B. Ashby, *Encyclopedia of Infectious Diseases* (New York: Facts On File, 1998); R. DeSalle and M. Brickman, "Infection: Introduction," in R. DeSalle, ed., *Epidemic! The World of Infectious Disease* (New York: New Press, 1999), pp. 79–83; J. Vallin, "The End of the Demographic Transition: Relief or Concern?" *Population and Development Review* 28, no. 1 (2002), pp. 105–120; B. Grun, *The Timetables of History* (New York: Simon & Schuster, 1982); J. N. Hays, *The Burdens of Disease: Epidemics and Human Response in Western History* (New Brunswick, NJ: Rutgers University Press, 2000); P. Ewald, "Portrait of a Pathogen," *Scientific American*, v. 276, no. 5 (1997), pp. 112–116; P. Ewald, *Plague Time: The New Germ Theory of Disease* (New York: Anchor Books, 2002); M. Oldstone, *Viruses, Plagues, and History* (New York: Oxford University Press, 1998); "New Mathematical Model Explains Changing Patterns in Epidemics," *World Disease Weekly* (February 13, 2000), p. NA; G. Garnett and E. Holmes, "The Ecology of Emergent Infectious Disease," *BioScience*, v. 46, no. 2 (1996), pp. 127–136; D. Arnold, "Smallpox and Colonial Medicine in Nineteenth Century India," in D. Arnold, ed., *Imperial Medicine and Indigenous Societies*, (New York: Manchester University Press, 1988), pp. 27–44; P. Hotez, "Dark Winters Ahead," *Foreign Policy* (November–December 2001), p. 84; G. Breu, "Unlike AIDS, Says a Historian, Ancient Plagues Swept the World Scythelike and Suddenly," *People Weekly*, v. 28 (1987), p. NA; M. Oldstone, *Viruses, Plagues, and History* (New York: Oxford University Press, 1998), p. 33; J. Longrigg, "Epidemic, Ideas and Classical Athenian Society," in T. Ranger and P. Slack, *Epidemics and Ideas: Essays on the Historical Perception of Pestilence*, (New York: Cambridge University Press, 1992), pp. 21–44; M. Matossian, *Poisons of the Past: Molds, Epidemics, and History* (New Haven, CT: Yale University Press, 1989); D. Childress, " 'Like Black Smoke': The Black Death's Journey," *Calliope*, v. 11 (2001) p. 7; R. Evans, "Epidemics and Revolutions: Cholera in Nineteenth Century Europe," in P. Slack, ed., *Epidemics and Ideas: Essays on the Historical Perception of Pestilence*, (New York: Cambridge University Press, 1992), p. 149–174; A. Crosby Jr., *The Columbian Exchange: Biological and Cultural Consequences of 1492* (Westport, CT: Greenwood Press, 1972); A. Ramenofsky, "Death by Disease," *Archaeology* (March/April 1992), pp. 47–49; J. Decker, "Depopulation of the Northern Plains Natives," *Social Science and Medicine*, 33, no. 4 (1991), pp. 381–393; N. Cook, "Sickness, Starvation, and Death in Early Hispaniola," *Journal of Interdisciplinary History*, v. 32, no. 3 (2002), pp. 349–386.
2. Africa's disease history is documented in J. Iliffe, *Africans: History of a Continent* (New York: Cambridge University Press, 1995); O. Ransford, *"Bid the Sickness Cease": Disease in the History of Black Africa* (London: John Murray, 1983).

3. For new diseases, see T. McMichael, *Human Frontiers, Environments, and Disease: Past Patterns, Uncertain Futures* (Cambridge: Cambridge University Press, 2001); L. Garrett, "Amplification," in DeSalle, ed., *Epidemic!*, p. 193; L. Garrett, *The Coming Plague* (New York: Farrar, Straus, and Giroux, 1994); World Health Organization, *World Health Report 2001* (Geneva, WHO: 2002), "Report on Global Surveillance of Epidemic-prone Infectious Diseases" (2000), "Fact Sheet Number 108, Epidemic Dysentery" (1996), "Dengue and Dengue Haemorrhagic Fever," Fact Sheet No. 117 (2002), and "Yellow Fever Fact Sheet" (2001); C. Ezzell, "It Came from the Deep: Scientists Warn of Outbreaks Stemming from the Ocean Abyss," *Scientific American*, 280, no. 6 (1999 at www.sciam.com); Turkington and Ashby, *Encyclopedia of Infectious Diseases*; C. Dye et al., "Erasing the World's Slow Strain: Strategies to Beat Multidrug-Resistant Tuberculosis," *Science*, 295 (2002), pp. 2042–2050; R. Lewis et al., "Timely Detection of Meningococcal Meningitis Epidemics in Africa," *The Lancet*, 358, no. 9278 (2001), p. 287; "Groups Forecast Epidemic," *Vaccine Weekly* (January 19, 2000), p. NA; J. Hooper, "A New Germ Theory," The Atlantic Monthly, v. 283, no.2 (1999), pp. 41–55; D. Heymann, "Controlling Epidemic Diseases," *World Health*, 49, no. 6 (1996), pp. 9–11; S. Hay et al., "Etiology of Interepidemic Periods of Mosquito-borne Disease," *Proceedings of the National Academy of Sciences*, 97, no. 16 (2000), pp. 9335–9339; R. Weiss, "Challenge for Humanity: War on Disease," *National Geographic* (February, 2002), pp. 5–31; "Cancer Boom," *Environmental Health Perspectives Supplements*, v. 102, no. 6–7 (June/July,1994), p. 516; American Public Health Association, "Infectious Disease Deaths Rise Despite Improved Detection" *The Nation's Health*, v. 28, no. 4 (1998), pp. 1–2 and "CDC Educates on Problem of Antimicrobial Resistance," *The Nation's Health*, v. 32, no. 4 (April, 2002), p. 4; P. Farmer, "Social Inequalities and Emerging Infectious Diseases," *Emerging Infectious Diseases*, v. 2, no. 4 (1996), pp. 259–269.
4. D. Narayan and G. Pennushi, *Poverty Trends and Voices of the Poor* (Washington, DC: World Bank Poverty Reduction and Economic Management Group, 1999), p. 33; on poverty, also see UN Development Program, *Human Development Report* (New York, NY: UNDP, 1997).
5. R. Weiss, "Challenge for Humanity: War on Disease," *National Geographic* (February, 2002), p. 12.

CHAPTER 5

1. For information on Social Darwinism, see P. Singer, *A Darwinian Left: Politics, Evolution and Cooperation* (New Haven, CT: Yale University Press, 1999); C. Zimmer, *Evolution: The Triumph of an Idea* (New York: HarperCollins, 2001), pp. 316–317; C. Reardon, "American Gothic: A New Curriculum Explores a Disturbing Side of the Progressive Era," *Teaching Tolerance*, no. 23 (Spring 2003), pp. 7–9.
2. Good Morning, Madam.

3. C. Cipolla, *Cristofano and the Plague: A Study in the History of Public Health in the Age of Galileo* (Berkeley: University of California Press, 1973), p. 61; A. Brandling-Bennett, "Our Long Struggle Against Epidemics," in R. DeSalle, ed., *Epidemic! The World of Infectious Disease* (New York: New Press, 1999), p. 160; F. Godolphin, *The Greek Historians*, v. 2, Thucydides Book 2, chaps. 47–52 (New York: Random House, 1942), p. 653; T. Zeldin, *An Intimate History of Humanity* (New York: HarperCollins, 1994), p. 123; S. Ell, "Plague and Leprosy in the Middle Ages: A Paradoxical Cross-Immunity?" *International Journal of Leprosy and Other Mycobacterial Diseases*, v. 55 (1987), pp. 345–350; D. Spoto, *Reluctant Saint: The Life of St. Francis of Assisi* (New York: Viking Compass, 2002); W. McNeill, *Plagues and Peoples* (Garden City, NY: Doubleday, 1976); B. Pullan, "Plague and perceptions of the poor in early modern Italy" in T. Ranger and P. Slack, eds., *Epidemics and Ideas: Essays on the Historical Perception of Pestilence* (Cambridge: Cambridge University Press, 1992), pp. 101–123; M. Dols, *The Black Death in the Middle East* (Princeton, NJ: Princeton University Press, 1977); L. Conrad, 1992, "Epidemic Disease in Formal and Popular Thought in Early Islamic Society," in T. Ranger and P. Slack, eds., *Epidemics and Ideas: Essays on the Historical Perception of Pestilence* (Cambridge: Cambridge University Press, 1992), pp. 77–100; D. Childress, "'Like Black Smoke': The Black Death's Journey," *Calliope*, v. 11, no. 7 (2001), p. 7; M. Jones and E. Rapley, "Behavioral Contagion and the Rise of Convent Education in France," *The Journal of Interdisciplinary History*, v. 31, no. 4 (2001), p. 489; R. Swenson, "Plagues, History, and AIDS," *American Scholar*, v. 51, no. 2 (2002), pp. 183–200; L. MacLehose, M. McKee, and J. Weinberg, "Responding to the Challenge of Communicable Disease in Europe," *Science*, v. 295 (March 15, 2002), pp. 2047–2050; A. Shively and J. Shively, "A Change Born of Death," *Calliope*, v. 11, no. 7 (2001), p. 24; M. Cowan, "A World Turned Upside Down," *Calliope*, v. 11, no. 7 (2001), p. 26; D. Feld, "The Church's Answer," *Calliope*, v. 11, no. 7 (2001), p. 20; D. Fox, "The Politics of Physicians' Responsibility in Epidemics: A Note on History," *The Hastings Center Report*, 18, no. 2 (1988), pp. S5–11; G. Lannom, "In the Words of the Survivors," *Calliope*, v. 11, no. 7 (2001) p. 9; A. Appleby, "The Disappearance of the Plague: A Continuing Puzzle," *The Economic History Review*, New Series, 33, no. 2 (1980), pp. 161–173; R. Evans, 1992, "Epidemics and Revolutions: Cholera in Nineteenth-century Europe," in T. Ranger and P. Slack, eds., *Epidemics and Ideas: Essays on the Historical Perception of Pestilence* (Cambridge: Cambridge University Press, 1992), pp. 149–173; A. Hardy, *The Epidemic Streets: Infectious Disease and the Rise of Preventive Medicine, 1856–1900* (Oxford: Clarendon Press, 1993); R. Chandavarkar, "Plague, Panic, and Epidemic Politics in India, 1896–1914," in T. Ranger and P. Slack, eds., *Epidemics and Ideas: Essays on the Historical Perception of Pestilence* (Cambridge: Cambridge University Press, 1992), pp. 203–240; R. De Salle, "Case Study: A Virus Comes to the Serengeti," in R. DeSalle, ed., *Epidemic! The World of Infectious* Disease (New York: New Press, 1999), pp. 10–11; M. Turshen, *The*

Political Ecology of Disease in Tanzania (New Brunswick, NJ: Rutgers University Press, 1984); D. Arnold, "Smallpox and Colonial Medicine in Nineteenth-century India," in D. Arnold, ed., *Imperial Medicine and Indigenous Societies* (New York: Manchester University Press, 1988), pp. 45–65; M. Worboys, "The Discovery of Colonial Malnutrition between the Wars," in D. Arnold, *Imperial Medicine and Indigenous Societies* (New York: Manchester University Press, 1988), pp. 208–225; Megan Vaughn, *Curing Their Ills: Colonial Power and African Illness* (Stanford, CA: Stanford University Press, 1991). For more on epidemic history, see notes 1 to 3 of chapter 4.

4. Opposing views on this question are presented by James Colgrove and Simon Szreter in the May 2002 issue of the *American Journal of Public Health*. See J. Colgrove, "The McKeown Thesis: A Historical Controversy and Its Enduring Influence" (pp. 725–729), and S. Szreter, "Rethinking McKeown: The Relationship Between Public Health and Social Change" (pp. 722–725).

CHAPTER 6

1. Edward Hopper recorded this speech in his wonderful book *The River: A Journey to the Source of HIV and AIDS* (Boston: Little, Brown, 1999).
2. P. Carmosino, "From Darwin to the Human Genome Project," 2002, at www.csuchico.edu; A. Brandt, *No Magic Bullet: A Social History of Venereal Disease in the United States since 1880* (New York: Oxford University Press, 1985).
3. Victorian sex can be studied in H. Horowitz, *Rereading Sex: Battles over Sexual Knowledge and Suppression in Nineteenth-Century America* (New York: Alfred A. Knopf, 2002); M. Sweet, *Inventing the Victorians: What We Think About Them and Why We're Wrong* (New York: St. Martin's Press, 2001); J. MacKenzie, *The Victorian Vision: Inventing New Britain* (London: V&A Publications, 2001).
4. References on STDs include the World Health Organization, *The World Health Report* (Geneva: WHO, 2001), pp. 144–145; C. Turkington and B. Ashby, *Encyclopedia of Infectious Diseases* (New York: Facts On File, 1998) under the headings of specific diseases; P. Ewald, *Plague Time: The New Germ Theory of Disease* (New York: Anchor Books, 2002); P. Ewald and G. Cochran, "Catching Up on What's Catching: Some Infections Are Slow to Be Recognized," *Natural History*, v. 108, no. 1 (1999), p. 46; R. DeSalle, ed., *Epidemic! The World of Infectious Disease* (New York: New Press, 1999); American Health Consultants, "Check STD Screening: Room for Improvement?" *Contraceptive Technology Update* (2003), p. 1; J. St. Lawrence et al., "STD Screening, Testing, Case Reporting, and Clinical and Partner Notification Practices: A National Survey of U.S. Physicians," *American Journal of Public Health*, 92, no. 11 (2002), pp. 1784–1788; M. Hogben et al., "Sexually Transmitted Disease Screening by United States Obstetricians and Gynecologists," *Obstetrics and Gynecology*, v. 100,

no. 4 (October, 2002), pp. 801–807; Centers for Disease Control, *Sexually Transmitted Disease Surveillance Report, 2001* (Atlanta: CDC, 2001); A. Crosby Jr., *The Columbian Exchange: Biological and Cultural Consequences of 1492* (Westport, CT: Greenwood Press, 1972); B. Hoff and C. Smith III, eds., *Mapping Epidemics: A Historical Atlas of Disease* (New York: Franklin Watts, 2000); E. Kolbert, "The Lost Mariner: The Self-Confidence that Kept Columbus Going Was His Undoing," *The New Yorker*, October 14–21, 2002, pp. 206–211; W. McNeill, "Unlike AIDS, Says a Historian, Ancient Plagues Swept the World Scythelike and Suddenly," *People Weekly*, 28 (1987); A. Speilman, 1999, "Emergence of New Diseases," in DeSalle, ed., *Epidemic!* pp. 19–22; S. Andreski, *Syphilis, Puritanism and Witch Hunts: Historical Explanations in Light of Medicine and Psychoanalysis with a Forecast about Aids* (New York: St. Martin's Press, 1989); S. Watts, *Epidemics and History: Disease, Power and Imperialism* (New Haven, CT: Yale University Press, 1997); A. Brandt, *No Magic Bullet* (New York: Oxford University Press, 1985); C. Quetel, *History of Syphilis* (Baltimore, MD: Johns Hopkins University Press, 1990); B. Wandrooij, "'The Thorns of Love': Sexuality, Syphilis and Social Control in Modern Italy," in R. Davidson and L. Hall, eds., *Sex, Sin and Suffering: Venereal Disease and European Society since 1870* (New York: Routledge, 2001), p. 139; "Roots of the Black Syphilis Epidemic in World War I," *New York Amsterdam News*, v. 88, no. 18 (1997), p. 13; J. Knowles, "Notes on the History of the Condom," Planned Parenthood Federation of America, 2003, www.plannedparenthood.org/articles/condomhistory.html; J. Cutler and R. Arnold, "Venereal Disease Control by Health Departments in the Past: Lessons for the Present," *American Journal of Public Health*, v. 78, no. 4 (1988), pp. 372–374; D. McBride, *From TB to AIDS: Epidemics among Urban Blacks Since 1900* (Albany: State University of New York Press, 1991); H. Dibble and D. Williams, "An Interview with Nurse Rivers" (pp. 321–339) and B. Roy, "The Tuskegee Syphilis Experiment: Biotechnology and the Administrative State" (pp. 299–320) in S. Reverby, *Tuskegee's Truths: Rethinking the Tuskegee Syphilis Study* (Chapel Hill: University of North Carolina Press, 2000); P. Levine, "Public Health, Venereal Disease and Colonial Medicine in the Later Nineteenth Century" (pp. 160–172) and K. MacPherson, "Health and Empire: Britain's National Campaign to Combat Venereal Diseases in Shanghai, Hong Kong and Singapore" (pp. 173–190) in R. Davidson and L. Hall, eds., *Sex, Sin and Suffering: Venereal Disease and European Society since 1870* (New York: Routledge, 2001); M. Vaughn, "Syphilis in Colonial East and Central Africa: The Social Construction of an Epidemic," in T. Ranger and P. Slack, eds., *Epidemics and Ideas: Essays on the Historical Perception of Pestilence* (Cambridge: Cambridge University Press, 1992), pp. 269–302; H. Wardlow, "Giving Birth to *Gonolia:* 'Culture' and Sexually Transmitted Disease among the Huli of Papua New Guinea," *Medical Anthropological Quarterly*, 16, no. 2 (2002), pp. 151–175.

CHAPTER 7

1. Ms. Lorch visited Uganda early in 1993. Her report on that experience hit the front page of the international edition of *The New York Times* on February 23, 1993.
2. For evolution, see A. Alland Jr., *Adaptation in Cultural Evolution: An Approach to Medical Anthropology* (New York: Columbia University Press, 1970), and references in other chapters.
3. For disease and evolution, see M. Grmek, *History of AIDS: Emergence and Origin of a Modern Pandemic* (Princeton, NJ: Princeton University Press, 1990); M. Specter, 2003, "The Vaccine: Has the Race to Save Africa from AIDS Put Western Science at Odds with Western Ethics?" *The New Yorker*, February 3, 2003, pp. 54–65; B. Levin et al., "Population Biology, Evolution, and Infectious Disease: Convergence and Synthesis," *Science*, v. 283 (1999), pp. 806–809; E. Alcamo, *AIDS in the Modern World* (Abingdon, UK: Blackwell Science, 2002); G. Garnett. and E. Holmes, "The Ecology of Emergent Infectious Diseases Pose an Ever-Emerging Threat to Humanity," *BioScience*, v. 46, no. 2 (1996), pp. 127–136; A. Read and L. Taylor, "The Ecology of Genetically Diverse Infections," *Science*, v. 292 (May 11, 2001), pp. 1099–1101; J. Lederberg, "Infectious Disease as an Example of Evolution," in R. DeSalle, ed., *Epidemic! The World of Infectious Disease*, (New York: New Press, 1999), pp. 13–17; J. Stephens et al., "Dating the Origin of the CCR5-Δ32 AIDS-Resistance Allele by the Coalescence of Haplotypes, *American Journal of Human Genetics*, v. 62 (1998): 1507–1515; A. Speilman, "Emergence of New Diseases," pp. 19–22 and M. Brickman, "Agents of Infection," pp. 43–49 in DeSalle, ed., *Epidemic! The World of Infectious Disease* (New York: New Press, 1999); H. Ochman and N. Moran, "Genes Lost and Genes Found: Evolution of Bacterial Pathogenesis and Symbiosis," *Science*, v. 202 (May 11, 2001), pp. 1096–1097; C. Zimmer, "*Wolbachia:* A Tale of Sex and Survival," *Science*, v. 292 (May 11, 2001), pp. 1093–1095; T. Clarke, "Bacteria Cause River Blindness: Microbes, Not the Worms that Carry Them, Aggravate the Immune System," *Nature Science Update*, Nature News Service (March 8, 2002, www.nature.com/nsu).
4. M. Small, *What's Love Got to Do with It? The Evolution of Human Mating* (New York: Bantam Doubleday Dell, 1995), p. 19.
5. Quote in Weiss, R., "Challenge for Humanity: War on Disease," *National Geographic* (February 2002), pp. 5–31.

CHAPTER 8

1. B. Davidson, *Africa: History of a Continent* (New York: Macmillan, 1966), p. 36.
2. For issues of globalization and economics, see R. Parker, "Administering the Epidemic: HIV/AIDS Policy, Models of Development, and International

Health," in L. Whiteford and L. Manderson, *Global Health Policy, Local Realities; The Fallacy of the Level Playing Field* (Boulder, CO: Lynne Reinner Publishers, 2001) p. 40; G. Soros, *George Soros on Globalization* (New York: Public Affairs Press, 2002); W. Finnegan, "Leasing the Rain: The World Is Running Out of Fresh Water, and the Fight to Control It Has Begun," *The New Yorker,* April 8, 2002, pp. 43–53; J. Sachs, "Helping the World's Poorest," *Economist,* v. 352 (August 14, 1999), p. 17.

3. S. Walsh and L. Rau, "Autoimmune Diseases: A Leading Cause of Death Among Young and Middle-Aged Women in the United States," *American Journal of Public Health,* v. 90, no. 9 (2000), pp. 1463–1466.

4. F. Fukuyama, "Is It All in the Genes?" *Commentary,* v. 104, no. 3 (1997), p. 30.

5. F. Sutton, "Development Ideology: Its Emergence and Decline," *Daedalus,* v. 118, no. 1 (Winter 1989), p. xi.

6. T. Bass, "Forgiveness Math," *Discover,* v. 14, no. 5 (1993), p. 62; C. Zimmer, *Evolution: The Triumph of an Idea* (New York: HarperCollins, 2002), pp. 248–253.

7. This phrase was coined by a Nigerian woman activist but has recently been picked up by the UN Special Envoy on AIDS, Stephen Lewis, and others.

8. L. Garrett, *Betrayal of Trust: The Collapse of Global Public Health* (New York: Hyperion, 2000).

9. P. Zeitz, *A Review of Experiences in Integrating an Expanded HIV/AIDS Response to the Debt Relief Process in Africa: 1999–2000,* and S. Ram et al., *A Summary of Resource Transfer Mechanisms.* Both publications were produced by the USAID-funded Synergy Project (www.synergyaids.com) for the UNAIDS workshop in Malawi entitled "Role of Debt Relief in Financing National HIV/AIDS Programs," November 2000.

Index